T0374883

Chronic Cardiac Care

A practical guide to specialist nurse management

Chronic Cardiac Care

A practical guide to specialist nurse management

Simon Stewart BA, BN, Grad Dip Ad Ed, PhD
Division of Health Sciences, University of South Australia, South Australia, and
Faculty of Health Sciences, University of Queensland, Queensland, Australia
Sally Inglis BN, BHSc (Hons)
Faculty of Health Sciences, University of Queensland, Queensland, Australia
Anna Hawkes BSc (Hons), MPH, PhD
Faculty of Health Sciences and Medicine, Bond University, Queensland, Australia

Foreword by
David R. Thompson

Blackwell
Publishing

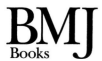

First edition 2006

1 2006

Library of Congress Cataloging-in-Publication Data
Stewart, Simon, 1964–
   Chronic cardiac care : a practical guide to specialist nurse management / Simon Stewart,
Sally Inglis, Anna Hawkes; foreword by David R. Thompson.
       p. ; cm.
   Includes bibliographical references and index.
   ISBN-13: 978-0-7279-1835-2 (alk. paper)
   ISBN-10: 0-7279-1835-4 (alk. paper)
   1. Heart—Diseases—Nursing.   2. Chronic diseases—Nursing.
   [DNLM: 1. Heart Diseases—nursing.   2. Chronic Disease—nursing.   3. Nursing
Care—standards.   WY 152.5 S851c 2006]   I. Inglis, Sally.   II. Hawkes, Anna.
III. Title.

   RC674.S84 2006
   616.1′20231—dc22

                                                                  2005031693

ISBN-13: 978-0-7279-1835-2
ISBN-10: 0-7279-1835-4

Set in 9.5/12 pt Meridien & Frutiger by TechBooks, New Delhi, India
Printed and bound in India by Replika Press Pvt. Ltd, Harayana

Commissioning Editor: Mary Banks
Editorial Assistant: Ariel Vernon
Development Editor: Nick Morgan
Production Controller: Debbie Wyer

For further information on Blackwell Publishing, visit our website:
http://www.blackwellpublishing.com

Contents

The privilege of travelling the globe and seeing first-hand so many wonderful cardiac programs, clinicians and researchers in action is tempered by my frequent absences from home. This book, therefore, is dedicated to my gorgeous wife Tania and beautiful daughters (big and small!) Laura Rose, Amy Rose and Sarah Niamh.

It is also dedicated to the "Heart of Soweto Study" research team, led by the inspirational Professor Karen Sliwa in Johannesburg, South Africa; may our collaboration be as long and fruitful!

Simon Stewart

Foreword

With the current focus of many clinical and research efforts and publications on acute coronary syndromes and the "hi-tech" aspects of modern cardiology, chronic cardiac care has received comparatively little attention. Yet, the combination of rapid advances in medical knowledge and technology, a progressively ageing population, and increased expectations from the public, including patients and families, and the health care professions demands that this neglected and important area of health care receives more attention. The number of people who have, or know someone who has, a chronic cardiac condition is enormous and older people are a particularly vulnerable and neglected group; the global impact in human and economic terms is alarming.

It is against this background that this book has been written. It covers the burden and management of chronic heart disease and much of the material presented draws on the clinical and research work of the first author, Simon Stewart, who has pioneered nurse-led, multidisciplinary, home-based interventions for patients with chronic heart failure. As he and his co-authors point out, many of the principles presented can be applied across different cardiac conditions, patient groups and professional boundaries. The book illustrates how innovative models of care, including outreach, can be organized and delivered. It also offers pointers to establishing a nurse-led program of chronic cardiac care and identifies a key role for the specialist cardiac nurse.

The book emphasizes the human aspects, often forgotten in many texts, and reminds the reader of the importance, where possible, of improving longevity and quality of life, but also accepting the reality that many of these patients will need optimal end-of-life care.

The authors are to be congratulated on producing a highly readable, topical, and succinct practical guide. I heartily (no pun intended) commend it as required reading to all those nurses working with patients with a chronic cardiac condition.

Professor David R. Thompson PhD FESC
Director, The Nethersole School of Nursing
The Chinese University of Hong Kong
September 2005

Preface

More than five years ago, my colleague Linda Blue and I published our first edition of a book that described the evolving evidence to support the widespread application of nurse-led, chronic heart failure management programs (Stewart S, Blue L (eds). *Improving outcomes in chronic heart failure with specialist nurse intervention: a practical guide*. London: BMJ Publishing Group, 2000). To say that we were overwhelmed by the response to this text would be an understatement. In a few short years we were able to publish a much more comprehensive and practical version of this book, based on an explosion of interest in the art and science of caring for patients with this truly malignant syndrome.

Unfortunately, the type of interest and effort dedicated to the management and care of patients with chronic heart failure has not been reciprocated in respect to the other common forms of chronic cardiac disease. Indeed, there has been an almost unhealthy focus on chronic heart failure-specific management to the exclusion of other debilitating and life-threatening disease states – even when present in the same patient! Clearly, within ageing western populations there are a growing number of older individuals who are suffering not only from chronic heart failure, but also from chronic angina pectoris, and chronic atrial fibrillation.

It is within this context that my colleagues and I present a text that examines a range of clinical issues (including the burden, treatment, and effective management) relating to optimizing health outcomes in chronic cardiac disease. As always, a workforce of specially trained nurses with the ability to work within the multidisciplinary, collaborative environment is clearly identified as the key to improving chronic cardiac care at the population level. There is little reason why the same principles applied to the effective management inherent to cardiac rehabilitation following an acute cardiac event, and chronic heart failure management programs, cannot be combined to deliver cost-effective cardiac care to those who qualify for neither form of management, but would benefit just the same.

This text, therefore, is an attempt to re-dress the imbalance in management programs targeting predominantly older patients with chronic cardiac disease. We certainly hope that the explosion of interest and evidence surrounding the specific management of chronic heart failure, with a dedicated role for specially qualified nurses, will be extended to those individuals unfortunate enough to suffer from other forms of chronic cardiac disease. It would certainly be gratifying to consider the wealth of new data and practical experiences available to fill an updated version of this text in a few years hence!

We certainly hope that you are able to use the information contained within this text to improve the level and effectiveness of chronic cardiac care within your own sphere of influence and practice.

Simon Stewart
December 2005

Section 1
Background

CHAPTER 1

Pathophysiology and epidemiologic burden of chronic cardiac disease

1.1 Introduction

Throughout the developed world there is an increasing realization that current health care systems are failing to cope with the twin demands imposed by ever-increasing expectations for more effective health care treatments (many of which would which be considered trivial or cosmetic in nature in past eras) for nonlethal conditions in relatively young individuals and, most significantly, the rising tide of older individuals who have survived previously fatal conditions only to succumb to a chronic disease that requires ongoing treatments. Both of these phenomena can be attributed to the rising affluence and sophistication of those fortunate enough to live in Western developed societies. The first of these demands is the product of a combination of more "disposable wealth", the desire to extend 'youthful' quality of life, and an increasing commercialization of medical and surgical therapies: any solution to this particular issue is well beyond the scope of this book! The second demand represents an inevitable trade-off between extended and more luxurious lifestyles with an increased risk of developing an "affluent disease" [1,2]. Significantly, in recent decades we have witnessed a historical watershed in human development with the declining impact of the traditional killers of malnourishment, infectious disease and violence on limited life expectancy, to a preponderance of "self-inflected" conditions that emerge in the latter years of an expanded life span [3,4]. Such a phenomenon has been exacerbated by advancing treatment options that merely prolong the inevitable in an ageing body rather than provide an "immortality elixir" that defies the natural ageing process once the inherent risks of being young are successfully navigated.

It is within this context that cardiovascular disease (typically comprising the combination cerebrovascular, cardiac, renovascular, and peripheral arterial disease) has become the single largest killer of humans in the world today [5]. Whilst all four of these closely related conditions are typically characterized by a narrowing of regional arteries (e.g. coronary or cerebral arteries) caused by the presence of atherosclerotic lesions and complicated by associated endothelial and platelet dysfunction and, frequently, metabolic abnormalities,

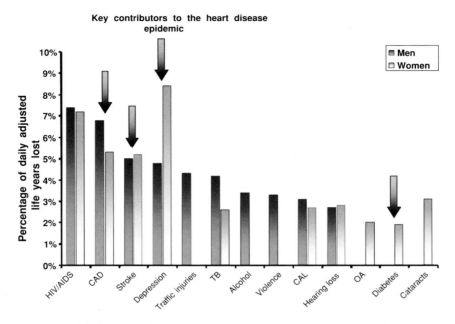

Figure 1.1 Global impact of the top ten causes of premature morbidity and mortality in men and women [5].

leading to a spectrum of conditions that reflect damage to the structural and functional integrity of affected organs (e.g. the heart, brain, or kidney), it is *chronic heart disease* that contributes most to premature morbidity and mortality in developed countries [1,2]. For example, Figure 1.1 shows the relative contributions of the top ten causes of healthy life years lost (expressed as disability-adjusted life years) in men and women on a global basis [5]. As will be discussed later in this chapter, the underlying nexus between heart disease and stroke, diabetes and depression cannot be overstated [6]. Moreover, there is an emerging relationship evident between heart disease and the human immune deficiency virus (HIV); particularly as individuals live longer with the virus and receive antiretroviral agents that may provoke the onset of coronary artery disease [7,8]. Even in developing countries, cardiovascular disease is responsible for 10% of premature disability/mortality and this figure is likely to rise with the adoption of more western-type lifestyles and prolonged exposure to HIV and its most effective treatment to date.

The three most common manifestations of chronic heart disease in Western developed countries and the major focus of this book, therefore, are as follows:
- Chronic angina pectoris.
- Chronic heart failure (CHF).
- Chronic atrial fibrillation (AF).

It is important to note that each of these distinct manifestations of chronic heart disease commonly coexist in the most advanced stages of the disease process (see below). They also dramatically impair the quality of life of affected individuals relative to age-matched controls and require continuous management to both minimize debilitating symptoms and reduce the probability of the following (often recurrent) events that mark a dramatic progression of the disease process or even the end of life:

- Acute coronary syndrome (e.g. acute myocardial infarction – AMI).
- Cerebrovascular event.
- Acute heart failure/cardiogenic shock.
- Sudden cardiac death (e.g. sustained ventricular fibrillation).

Figure 1.2 shows the typical progression of the disease process in high-risk individuals who initially survive an acute cardiac event and subsequently develop chronic cardiac disease; the likelihood of developing chronic angina pectoris, heart failure and atrial fibrillation increasing sequentially during the fourth and fifth, sixth and seventh and eighth and ninth decades of life, respectively, for each of these conditions. From a societal perspective, affected individuals consume the largest component of health care expenditure via the combination of chronic treatment and, more importantly, extremely costly procedures and recurrent/prolonged hospital stay.

This introductory chapter summarizes the key features of the most common manifestations of chronic cardiac disease in respect to: (i) the common pathways and risk factors preceding the development of underlying heart disease, (ii) the specific pathophysiologic mechanisms that underpin typical signs and symptoms associated with the three most common, chronic manifestations of heart disease, and (iii) the epidemiologic burden imposed by each condition (both on an individual and societal level).

1.2 Risk factors: the common pathways to chronic cardiac disease

Anyone approaching the rising burden imposed by chronic cardiac disease from a fatalistic perspective might be tempted to merely plot the rising tide of emerging cases and deal with consequences (i.e. apply cost-effective disease management programs to limit hospital use) without attempting to understand the reasons behind the epidemic. In one sense, the most powerful factor driving the enormous pressure on health care systems of developed countries around the world is the progressive ageing of the population. Naturally, this paradoxical side-effect of the combination of improved living standards, public health initiatives and specific health care interventions (e.g. reperfusion therapies for AMI) is one that will be tolerated by any society. Alternatively, it does make sense to either totally prevent (an extremely difficult task even with modern-day treatments) or delay the onset of chronic cardiac disease; hence the importance of primary prevention strategies. Clearly this is *not* the focus of this book. However, the importance of so-called "secondary prevention"

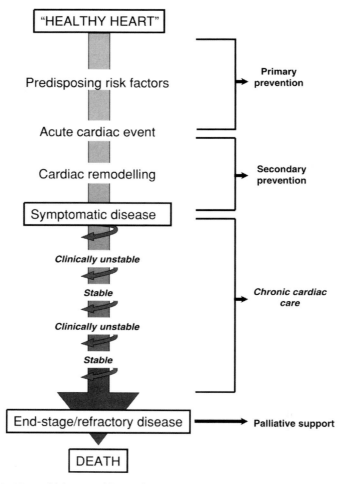

Figure 1.2 'Natural history' of heart disease in adult men and women living in Western developed countries.

(i.e. addressing risk factors after a diagnosis of heart disease is established) is often overlooked in the context of an older individual with a chronic man-ifestation of their heart disease as opposed to the younger individual who has survived an acute cardiac event without apparent residual effects. As sug-gested by Figure 1.2, whilst it is desirable to prevent a secondary event in the latter, it is often as important to slow the progression of heart disease (and therefore the time to third, fourth, or fifth cardiac events) to improve quality of life, reduce costly morbid events, and prolong survival by addressing the "fuels" (in this case modifiable risk factors and contributory causes) that drive the underlying pathological processes of the disease.

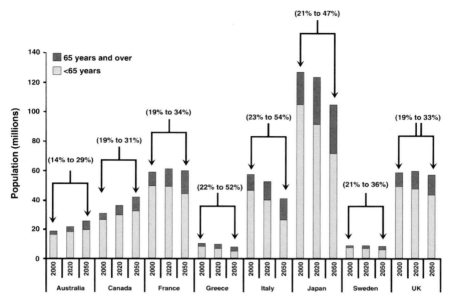

Figure 1.3 The progressive ageing of Western developed countries [9].

Ageing societies: chronic cardiac disease

As demonstrated by Figure 1.3, almost every developed country, irrespective of whether it expected to increase or decrease in its overall size, is progressively ageing with the proportion of men and women aged 65 years or more increasing dramatically [9]. For example, in the United States the total population is predicted to rise from 244 million to 274 million during the period of 2000 to 2050 (a 13% increase) [9]. Significantly the proportion of men and women aged 65 years or more will increase by 117%, the proportion of the population in this age group rising from 14% to 28% – an absolute increase of 40 million people [9]. These figures are largely due to the flow-on effect of the postwar "Baby Boomers" who are now reaching old age. In the past, western societies have been able to afford the care of older individuals because of the preponderance of younger individuals who actively contribute to wealth generation and tax revenues. However, as shown by Figure 1.3, due to progressively falling fertility rates, the ratio of relatively young and healthy individuals versus older individuals at risk of chronic illness is dramatically changing.

Figure 1.4, which summarizes data from a contemporary study of four coronary heart disease registers in London, United Kingdom [10], demonstrates the overwhelming significance of an ageing population on health care services. This study examined the prevalence of clinically manifest (e.g. those with chronic angina pectoris) and asymptomatic (e.g. where optimal treatment had been applied) cases of coronary heart disease in a population cohort of 378,021 men and women in 2000/2001. The overall, age-adjusted prevalence

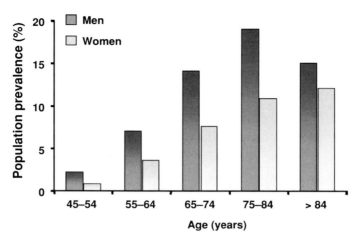

Figure 1.4 Proportion of men and women affected by coronary heart disease in a large population cohort in the UK: a clear age-related gradient in cases [10].

of coronary heart disease in this large population cohort was 7.8% in men (95% CI 7.6 to 8.3%) and 4.2% in women (95% CI 4.0 to 4.3%) [10]. Significantly, less than 2% of men and women aged 45–54 years combined were diagnosed with the disease [10]. This figure rose dramatically (10–15 fold) in those individuals who had reached the age of 65 years or more [10]. Due to the accumulative effects of a lifetime of use and, in western societies in particular, abuse of the heart, age is the most *powerful* and nonmodifiable predictor of heart disease.

Overall, more men than women are affected by coronary heart disease, but when examining the total burden of symptomatic heart disease, this gender gap narrows. Although women are more likely to develop symptomatic or fatal heart disease at a later stage in their life (they lag approximately 10 years behind men in respect to the age-adjusted risk of developing a symptomatic form of the disease after the age of 40 years [11]) their more advanced age leaves them more susceptible to chronic forms of the heart disease. This is particularly true, if their chronic condition arises from less life-threatening conditions such as hypertension and/or diabetes.

Modifiable risk factors: key targets for intervention in chronic cardiac disease

Once an individual has been diagnosed with a chronic form of heart disease, there is a range of risk factors that can be considered as "nonmodifiable" (over and above age and a positive family history suggesting a genetic component [12]) at this late stage of the disease progression and, therefore, cannot be considered for active intervention. Such factors may include the following:

- Socioeconomic deprivation (particularly from an early age) [13].
- Infection leading to structural cardiac abnormalities (e.g. rheumatic heart disease) or contributes to an overall inflammatory state that may contribute

to atherosclerosis and platelet activation: hence the increasing interest in the predictive value of elevated C-reactive protein [14,15].
- Congenital abnormalities that may not have been corrected at an early age and therefore may have led to ventricular remodeling and/or valvular abnormalities [16].
- Poor nutritional patterns (e.g. leading to prolonged hyperhomocystinemia due to lack of a vegetable-rich diet) [17].
- A past traumatic event leading to psychological distress [18].

Alternatively, there are a number of major modifiable risk-factors (both directly causal and strongly associated with the development of the disease) that, if still "active" in an individual with chronic cardiac disease should be carefully assessed and considered for active intervention – even if their risk factor profile is borderline. The five major risk factors that both contribute and continue to exacerbate an epidemic of chronic heart disease are as follows:

1 *Smoking tobacco (both inhaled and passive)*. This is the single most important target for heart disease prevention around the globe. Case-fatality rates for cardiovascular disease are more than double in smokers with a disproportionate number of premature life-years lost. The "contaminated" smoke from cigarettes includes ammonia, benzene, carbon monoxide, and nicotine and is linked to tachycardia, vasoconstriction, hypoxia, and atherogenesis [19].

2 *Abnormal lipid profile*. The link between dietary cholesterol and CAD has long been known and confirmed by large-scale population studies [20–22]. Initial fatty streaks and lipid recruitment into atherosclerotic lesions in the coronary arteries are a key process in the development of coronary heart disease. It is on this basis that HMG-CoA reductase inhibitors commonly referred to as the "statins", are now routinely used to normalize the lipid profile of both at risk individuals [23] and those with established coronary heart disease [24,25]. As will be outlined in Chapter 2, rather than concentrate on overall cholesterol/ or blood fat (triglyceride) levels there are clear differential targets to optimize the lipid profile of at-risk individuals. For example, the Helsinki Heart Study found a threefold increased risk of cardiac events in subjects with a high LDL-HDL cholesterol ratio and triglyceride levels greater than 200 mg/dL [22]. As such, LDL cholesterol is a particularly atherogenic lipoprotein whilst HDL is antiatherogenic [26]. Apolipoproteins also play an important role in the initial development of atherosclerosis and the progression of the underlying disease [27]. In the recent Apolipoprotein-related Mortality Risk (AMORIS) Study of 175,553 men and women, followed-up for approximately 5.5 years, the risk of an acute myocardial infarction was highest in those with the worst versus most optimal ApoB: ApoA-I ratio (4.8-fold for men and 4.0-fold for women) [28].

3 *Hypertension*. Along with an abnormal lipid profile and smoking, hypertension (both systolic and diastolic) forms part of the traditional "triad" of the primary prevention of heart disease. A highly prevalent condition (the American Heart Association estimates that 50 million individuals in

the United States and 1 billion worldwide are affected) [29], hypertension greatly increases the risk of developing cardiovascular disease. Population-based studies show a consistent relationship between higher blood pressure values and higher risk for developing all forms of cardiovascular disease: for individuals aged 40–70 years, each increment of 20 mmHg in systolic and 10 mmHg in diastolic blood pressure doubles the risk of disease across the entire blood pressure range [30].

4 *Diabetes/metabolic abnormalities.* It is estimated that more than 2% of the world's population have diabetes and this figure will double by 2025 [28]. In Europe and North America the prevalence of diabetes and its most common form (Type II Diabetes) is particularly high – approximately 4% and rising [29]. The number of adults with either high fasting glucose levels and/or impaired glucose tolerance is also rising in parallel to high-fat/carbohydrate diets, obesity and sedentary lifestyles. Significantly, the triad of hypertriglyceridemia, low HDL cholesterol levels, and elevated levels of LDL cholesterol particles is common in both a prediabetic state (the so-called Metabolic Syndrome) and established adult-onset Type-II diabetes. [31]. Insulin resistance is also closely associated with endothelial and platelet dysfunction. In the United States, 17% of men and 15% of women aged 60 years or more are diagnosed with this condition [28].

5 *Obesity.* The World Health Organisation definition for overweight is a body mass index (BMI) of >25 kg/m^2 and obesity when this threshold reaches >30 kg/m^2 [5]. In most affluent countries the prevalence of overweight individuals is increasing dramatically with approximately 40% of the adult population affected [5]. Typical of western countries, the British Heart Foundation recently estimated that the number of obese adults in that country has doubled in the last decade from 14% to 22%. [32]. Amongst "Baby Boomers" aged 40–59 in the United States, a startling 75% of men and 65% of women are overweight [28]. The proportion of overweight children was also estimated to be approximately 25% [29]. Men and women with a waist circumference of >90 cm (35 inches) and 100 cm (40 inches), respectively, are at particular risk for cardiovascular disease [29]. Not surprisingly, obesity is closely linked to an abnormal lipid profile, insulin resistance/diabetes, and hypertension [33].

The importance of targeting these risk factors, even if they appear to be borderline, is best illustrated by data from the NHANES III survey of 681 men and 807 women living in the United States: Figure 1.5 (adapted from original data) [34] shows the risk profile of these subjects according to whether they had an "optimal" profile, a borderline risk or established risk for coronary heart disease in relation to their blood pressure, lipid profile, glucose tolerance and smoking history. Overall, 26% of men and 41% of women had at least one borderline risk factor [34]. However, isolated borderline risk factors (i.e. those in the absence of high risk factors) accounted for only 10% of age-adjusted, 10-year coronary heart disease events. The presence of borderline risk factors in the presence of established risk factor thresholds increase the

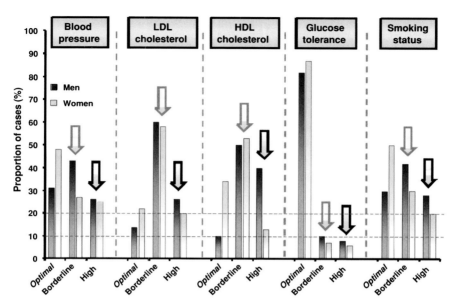

Figure 1.5 Risk factor profile of a large representative cohort of adult men and women living in the United States [34].

risk of coronary heart disease events incrementally. For example, the presence of one "high" risk factor in men conveyed a 2.73% risk of a coronary heart disease event within 10 years overall (all ages). The presence of two, three, or four borderline risk factors increased this risk to 5.31%, 8.05%, and 14.46%, respectively [34]. There is no evidence to suggest that "borderline" risk factors are any less important in secondary prevention in the context of preestablished chronic cardiac disease.

There are, of course, a range of other positive and negative factors that have the potential to both increase influence the risk of developing heart disease and modulate its severity once a chronic, symptomatic form of the disease has developed. These include:

- *Exercise.* The benefits of exercise in improving general cardiovascular fitness (e.g. lower resting heart rate and blood pressure), reducing weight, reducing blood sugar and cholesterol levels in addition to improving endothelial/platelet function are well known. [35]. However, in affluent countries, only one-third of the population moderately exercise for the recommended 30 minutes, five times per week [29,32].
- *Vegetables and vitamin B.* Homocysteine is a metabolite of an essential amino acid which can only enter the body via ingested food (predominantly animal protein). In population studies, elevated homocysteine levels have been shown to be independently associated with cardiovascular outcomes due to platelet activation, endothelial function, and atherogenesis [17]. For

example in an elderly cohort of subject from Framingham, the adjusted relative risk for cardiovascular mortality in those with the upper quartile of serum homocysteine levels was 1.54 (95% CI, 1.31–1.82) compared to those with the lowest concentrations [36]. Significantly, folate, which is required for the metabolism of homocysteine is predominantly derived from vegetables. Risk minimization, therefore, involves a vegetable rich diet, less meat and/or supplements of folic acid and B vitamins.

- *Stress and psychological status.* In recent years there has been increasing recognition of the importance of stress and other psychosocial factors such as depression in the development of heart disease [37]. Expert groups have concluded that there is "strong and consistent evidence of an independent causal association between depression, social isolation and lack of quality social support and the causes and consequences of heart disease" [38]. In support of this, the INTERHEART Study (see below) [39] found that psychosocial factors (as measured by four simple questions about stress at work and home, financial stress and major life events in the past year) independently predicted the risk of AMI [39].
- *Socioeconomic deprivation.* There is also increasing recognition that equitable access to health foods, "healthy" messages, healthier lifestyle choices (e.g. safe areas to exercise) and optimal health care will reduce the risk and consequences of heart disease [40,41]. Population studies consistently demonstrate that individuals from lower socioeconomic circumstances have a worse risk factor profile and outcomes than their more affluent counterparts [42–44].

Figure 1.6 summarizes data from the INTERHEART Study [39] which examined the overall epidemiologic importance of both negative and positive factors (as expressed by each factor's population attributable risk*) in determining the incidence of one of the most important markers of chronic cardiac disease – nonfatal, AMI. It is important to note that the INTERHEART Study was a large, international, standardized case control study of similar cohorts in 52 countries. During the study 262 centers recruited men and women with a first-ever AMI and presenting to their local coronary care unit. At least one age and sex-matched control was recruited for each case: a total of 12,461 cases and 14,637 controls were recruited overall [39].

As discussed in the introduction of this chapter, the progressive ageing and risk factor profile of western societies in particular has led to an inevitable epidemic of heart disease. Before reviewing the extent of the burden imposed

---

Population attributable risk. This can be defined as the product of the absolute risk of developing a disease for any given risk factor by the proportion of people affected, it provides a measure of what proportion of that disease may be avoided by eliminating/ minimizing that risk factor. For example, a risk factor that imparts a very low attributable risk (i.e. a 10% increased risk) for any given disease state will have a larger population attributable risk if it is much more prevalent in the community than a more "potent" risk factor (i.e. a 200% or two-fold increased risk) that affects only a small minority.

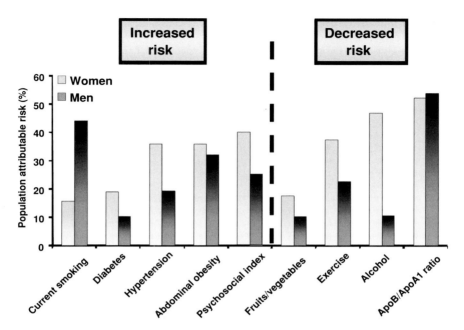

Figure 1.6 Population attributable risk of "positive" and "negative" risk factors for the development of coronary heart disease and subsequently chronic heart disease in the INTERHEART Study [39].

by this epidemic, it is appropriate to firstly review the pathological mechanisms that turn the potent "cocktail" of progressively ageing populations and highly prevalent risk factors into the current problems confronting health care systems around the globe.

1.3 Underlying pathophysiology and consequences of the most common manifestations of chronic cardiac disease

Defining and classifying chronic angina pectoris

One of the most common and debilitating manifestations of ischemic heart disease is angina pectoris. Angina pectoris, a clinical syndrome, indicates an imbalance between myocardial oxygen supply and demand, the cause of which is often atherosclerotic disease of the coronary arteries leading to a narrowing of the vessel lumen and subsequent reduction in blood supply [45]. Angina is characterized by pain or discomfort in the chest, jaw, shoulder, back, or arm and is often precipitated by exertion or emotional stress and usually relieved by nitroglycerine or rest [46].

The terms *chronic or stable* angina may be used to describe anginal symptoms which have occurred over several weeks without major deterioration [47].

Table 1.1 Canadian Classification of Angina [53].

Functional class	Descriptor
Class I	"Ordinary physical activity does not cause angina" for example walking or climbing stairs, angina occurs with strenuous or rapid or prolonged exertion.
Class II	"Slight limitation of ordinary activity" for example, angina occurs walking, climbing stairs, after meals, in cold, under emotional stress, the first few hours after waking, walking more than two blocks on level surface, or climbing more than one flight of ordinary stairs at a normal pace and in normal conditions.
Class III	"Marked limitation of ordinary physical activity" for example angina occurs walking one or two blocks on level surface or climbing one flight of stairs in normal conditions at a normal pace.
Class IV	"Inability to carry on any physical activity without discomfort – angina syndrome may be present at rest."

Furthermore to distinguish chronic angina, the episodes are repetitive over months or years and the symptoms are reversible [48].

The most severe and debilitating form of chronic angina is chronic refractory angina, which has been estimated to affect 10–15% of all patients with chronic angina [49]. Chronic refractory angina may be defined as angina which persists despite a combination of both pharmacologic and revascularization procedures, leaving the patient with residual deficits in myocardial perfusion [49,50] due to underlying coronary heart disease. The patient with chronic refractory angina experiences a diminished quality of life due to recurrent episodes of angina, lack of energy, poor sleeping patterns, decreased physical capacity and increased prevalence of anxiety and depression [51,52].

The functional impairment associated with this syndrome is often classified according to the Canadian Cardiovascular Society Classification of Angina – see Table 1.1 [53]. Beyond this fairly straightforward classification system, in clinical practice it is imperative to comprehensively assess the location of the discomfort, its relationship to exercise, character, and duration [47]. Any suspicion of the presence of unstable angina pectoris requires urgent medical assessment and treatment. This form of angina is defined by ESC as: an acute coronary syndrome, and "is said to be unstable if preexisting angina worsens abruptly for no apparent reason or when new angina develops at a relatively low work load or at rest" [47]. Unstable angina has been further classified by ESC as "prolonged (>20 mins) anginal pain at rest, new onset (*de novo*) severe (Class III of Canadian Cardiovascular Society Classification – see Table 1.1) angina or recent destabilization of previously stable angina with at least Canadian Cardiovascular Society Classification III angina characteristics" [54].

Table 1.2 Rose definition of angina (adapted from the original [55]).

Angina	A chest pain or discomfort with the following characteristics: a) The site must include the sternum *or* the left arm and left anterior chest b) It must be provoked by either hurrying or walking uphill (or walking on level ground if that is all the person can normally achieve) c) When it occurs on walking, it must make the person stop, or slow their pace, unless nitroglycerin is taken d) It must disappear on the majority of occasions within 10 minutes or less when the person stops and rests
Possible Myocardial Infarction	"One or more attacks of severe pain across the front of the chest lasting for 30 minutes or longer"

The Rose Angina Questionnaire [55] also relates the diagnosis of angina to functional capacity, but in its original form does not stratify patients into classes according to their functional capacity. As can be seen from Table 1.2, it facilitates the differentiation of anginal pain with other causes of chest pain (see Table 1.2). It defines angina as chest pain which limits exertion and is located over the sternum, or the left chest of left arm and is relieved by rest within 10 minutes [55]. This differs from the less distinctive pain relating to myocardial infarction (see Table 1.2) [55].

Prinzmetal, or variant angina, is another form of acute angina that is characterized by transient episodes of acute myocardial ischemia, with or without chest pain, and is often associated with transient ST segment elevation seen on ECG, which may last several minutes and resolve spontaneously or following administration of nitroglycerin [54]. It is important to note that *chronic angina pectoris* will be the focus of this discussion rather than those forms of angina which fall under the umbrella of acute coronary syndromes (e.g. unstable angina, Prinzmetal angina, and most significantly, AMI).

Pathogenesis of chronic angina pectoris

There are many contributing and causal factors in the development of chronic angina pectoris. For the purposes of this text we will consider angina as pain and discomfort due to myocardial ischemia associated with coronary artery disease. It is recognized that angina may be present in subjects with other cardiac conditions, such as aortic stenosis, uncontrolled hypertension, hypertrophic cardiomyopathy, and valvular heart disease and may be present in those with normal coronary arteries and myocardial ischemia related to spasm or endothelial dysfunction [46]. Whilst these other pathologies should not be overlooked by the clinician they are outside the scope of this text.

Angina occurs when there is insufficient blood flow to a region of the myocardium, leading to an imbalance between myocardial oxygen supply and

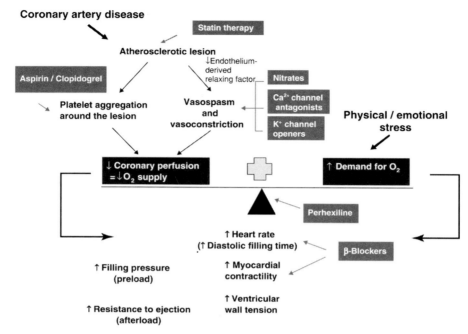

Figure 1.7 The mismatch between supply and demand for oxygen in chronic angina pectoris.

demand (see Figure 1.7) [45], this disparity gives rise to metabolic changes within the myocardium and impacts cardiac efficiency [56]. Insufficiency of blood flow to the myocardium is multifactorial; however, atherosclerotic disease of the coronary arteries is invariably the cause [47].

Atherosclerotic disease of the vessels often begins with the development of precursors of advanced lesions which may cause ischaemic heart disease. The initial lesion is type I, representing very early changes – an increase in the number of macrophages within the intima (inner most layer of an artery wall) and the appearance of foam cells (macrophages filled with lipid droplets) [57]. Type II lesions are also known as "fatty streaks", composed of lipid rich macrophages and T lymphocytes deposited within the intima [58]. These "fatty streaks" considered to precede the development of intermediate atherosclerotic lesions, [57] develop in childhood [59]. Kavey et al. [60] states that:

> "pathological studies have shown that both the presence and extent of atherosclerotic lesions at autopsy after unexpected death of children and young adults correlate positively and significantly with established risk factors namely low-density lipoprotein cholesterol, triglycerides, systolic and diastolic blood pressure, body mass index and presence of smoking".

Type III lesions, also known as intermediate lesions are those which form a morphological and chemical bridge between the precursor lesions (type I and II) and more advanced lesion such as an atheroma (type IV) [57]. These intermediate or preatheroma lesions are composed of macrophages, smooth muscle cells [58] and extracellular lipid droplets [57]. Overtime this extracellular lipid of the type III lesion develops into a lipid core marking the transition to a type IV lesion or atheroma [61]. Around the *fourth decade* of life atheromas may develop thick fibrous layers of connective tissue, indicative of the type V lesion or fibroatheroma. Furthermore these lesions may fissure, develop a hematoma or thrombus and are then classified as type VI [61]. It is the rupture or fissure of these fibrous lesions leading to hemorrhage, thrombosis, and complete occlusion of the artery which precipitates an acute coronary event [62]. As such, "morbidity and mortality from atherosclerosis is largely due to type IV and type V lesions in which disruptions of the lesions surface, hematoma or hemorrhage, and thrombotic deposits have developed" [61].

Several theories debate the causal factor in the initial development of a atherosclerotic plaque and its most common sequale – coronary heart disease. The most accepted theory being the "response to injury hypothesis", which hypothesizes that endothelial injury may lead to an "excessive inflammatory-fibroproliferative response" [58]. It has been reported that not only is the reduction in the diameter of the lumen important in terms of blood flow, but also the length and the number of stenoses present within the vessel [47], and that in the case of chronic angina pectoris one or more obstructions in the major coronary arteries is usually present, often with greater than 70 per cent narrowing of the diameter of the lumen [48].

A recurrent episode of chronic angina is often, but not always, initiated by a demand for increased myocardial blood flow [48]. Physical exertion or emotional stress can cause changes in the tone of the coronary vessels, subsequently altering the luminal diameter of an atherosclerotic area of the vessel due to smooth muscle constriction or dilatation [47], leading to angina. The resulting ischemia initiates a cascade of physiological processes, facilitated by the endocrine and nervous systems, such as tachycardia, shortened diastolic filling time, and coronary vasoconstriction [47]. Due to the subsequent increased blood pressure and tachycardia there is even greater demand for blood flow to the myocardium [47].

During an episode of angina, the limitation of myocardial blood flow leads to a shift in metabolism within the cardiac tissue and accumulation of metabolic byproducts, impacting the functioning of the myocardium [56]. Normal cardiac metabolism involves the oxidation of free fatty acids (60–90%), comprising mainly of long chain fatty acids, with the balance derived from the metabolism of lactate and glucose [63,64]. Long chain fatty acids are transported into myocyte cytoplasm via several enzymes [65], whereupon they become bound to binding proteins and are activated to long-chain acyl CoA [66]. Entry into the mitochondria, the site of energy production is via the action of carnitine-palmitoyl-transferase I and II (CPT-I, CPT-II) [65]. β-oxidation occurs within the mitochondria generating acetyl-CoA, which enters the tricarboxylic acid cycle and leads to the formation of adenosine triphosphate (ATP) [65]. During ischemia, metabolic adaptations occur mimicking those of

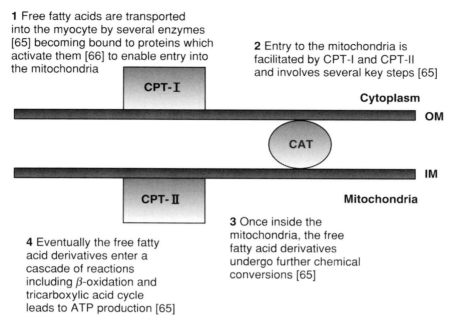

1 Free fatty acids are transported into the myocyte by several enzymes [65] becoming bound to proteins which activate them [66] to enable entry into the mitochondria

CPT-I

2 Entry to the mitochondria is facilitated by CPT-I and CPT-II and involves several key steps [65]

Cytoplasm

OM

CAT

IM

CPT-II

Mitochondria

4 Eventually the free fatty acid derivatives enter a cascade of reactions including β-oxidation and tricarboxylic acid cycle leads to ATP production [65]

3 Once inside the mitochondria, the free fatty acid derivatives undergo further chemical conversions [65]

Figure 1.8 Normal cardiac metabolic pathways.

the fetal heart by shifting substrate selection to glucose metabolism [65]. This is considered an advantage, although the oxidation of free fatty acids yields more ATP per gram of substrate, it occurs at the expense of greater oxygen consumption [65]. Fatty acids require 10–15% more oxygen to generate an equivalent amount of ATP as glucose metabolism [67]. However, despite some alterations in metabolism during ischemia, the oxidation of free fatty acids continues to be the predominant substrate [68]. Not only does this continued oxidation of free fatty acids expend the limited supply of oxygen, but also the continued uptake of free fatty acids and catabolism during ischemia gives rise to dysfunction of the myocardium [69]. Glucose oxidation is suppressed by the high rate of free fatty acid oxidation, via a direct inhibitory action on pyruvate dehydrogenase [70] which leads to proton and lactate accumulation in the ischemic myocyte precipitating a cascade of biochemical dysfunction such as a decreased intracellular pH and loss of calcium homeostasis, resulting in the impairment of myocardial contractility [64]. Cardiac efficiency is decreased by this process as energy is diverted to the restoration of intracellular homeostasis rather than myocyte contraction [65] (see Figure 1.8).

Pathophysiologic consequences of chronic angina pectoris

Not only is chronic angina a debilitating condition which impacts on quality of life, but it also places the patient at risk of developing several other clinically important sequale. Patients with chronic angina are at an elevated risk of developing further complications of coronary disease such as AMI, CHF, AF, and noncardiac vascular events such as stroke [71]. Given the likely presence of atherosclerosis within the vasculature the patient is at risk of experiencing an acute coronary event, precipitated by the rupture, hemorrhage, thrombosis and embolism of a preexisting atheroma leading to unstable angina or irreversible myocardial ischemia [48], which may or may not be fatal. The development of an AMI and a subsequent mural thrombus and embolism may lead to a cerebrovascular event such as a stroke. Chronic, long-term ischemia of the myocardium as occurs in chronic angina can lead to impairment of contractile function, precipitating the development of CHF [72] and the beginning of further decline in the patient's prognosis and day-to-day living. The patient is also at an increased risk of developing serious and potentially life-threatening arrhythmias [73].

Chronic angina pectoris is a condition for which the true burden is represented not only by fatal events, such as the development of AMI or sudden cardiac death, but by the hospitalisation of these patients for both coronary and non-coronary events.[74]. Unfortunately very few population-based studies have examined the long-term consequences of angina. A 20-year follow-up of the Renfrew/Paisley cohort in the West of Scotland [74] provides an outline of the long-term consequences of angina. At 20 years, for the cohort of middle-aged men and women with angina at baseline (10% of the total cohort) the following findings were reported:

- A case fatality rate of 67.7% in men and 43.3% in women compared to those without angina, 45.4% and 30.4% respectively.
- Men had an increased adjusted relative risk of cardiovascular death or hospitalization (RR 1.62), AMI (RR 1.80) and CHF (RR 1.62) relative to those without angina.
- Women also experienced increased adjusted risk of death or hospitalization (RR 1.48), AMI (RR 1.67) and CHF (RR 2.05) relative to those without angina.

It has been suggested that relative to other cardiac conditions chronic angina pectoris has a good prognosis in the majority of patients [47]; however, studies such as the Renfrew/Paisley follow-up [74] and others [71,75,76] which have examined the long-term prognosis of those with this symptomatic form of coronary heart disease have indicated that it is associated with an increased risk relative to those without angina of both cardiac morbidity and mortality.

Not only are patients with chronic angina at risk of developing other cardiac conditions but the condition itself also impacts significantly on the patient's life. Chronic angina and especially refractory angina may decrease a patient's quality of life through impairment of standard physical activities and may require an adjustment to the patient's normal lifestyle. Such patients are also at increased risk of depression and anxiety [51,52].

Defining and classifying chronic heart failure

Most clinicians would immediately recognize chronic heart failure (CHF) as a disabling and deadly condition that typically represents the end product of a lifetime of "insults" to the structural integrity and efficiency of the heart.

Table 1.3 An evolving definition of chronic heart failure.

Source	Definition
Wood (1968)	"A state in which the heart fails to maintain an adequate circulation for the needs of the body despite a satisfactory venous filling pressure" [77]
Braunwald (1992)	"A state in which an abnormality of cardiac function is responsible for failure of the heart to pump blood at a rate commensurate with the requirements of the metabolising tissues or, to do so, only from an elevated filling pressure" [78]
Packer (1988)	"A complex clinical syndrome characterised by abnormalities of left ventricular function and neurohormonal regulation which are accompanied by effort intolerance, fluid retention and reduced longevity" [79]
Poole-Wilson (1985)	"A clinical syndrome caused by an abnormality of the heart and recognised by a characteristic pattern of haemodynamic, renal, neural and hormonal responses" [80]
AHA/ACC (2001)	"Heart Failure is a complex clinical syndrome that can result from any structural or functional cardiac disorder that impairs the ability of the ventricle to fill with or eject blood" [81]
ESC (2005)	"A syndrome in which the patients should have the following features: symptoms of heart failure, typically breathlessness or fatigue, whether at rest or during exertion or ankle swelling and objective evidence of cardiac dysfunction at rest" [82].

However, given that CHF is a syndrome encompassing a complex pathological process that is the terminal manifestation of a number of diverse but often interrelated cardiac disease states (including coronary heart disease, chronic systolic hypertension and in an ageing population, chronic AF) and a broad spectrum of clinical presentations, it is not easy to define. Table 1.3 provides a list of the more recognized and quoted definitions of CHF with a progressive emphasis on the inability of the heart's ability to pump, the role of the neuroendocrine activation, a system-wide failure (e.g. renal, respiratory and skeletal muscle dysfunction) the clinical aspects of the syndrome and, more latterly, the need to establish an underlying cardiac pathology (even in the presence of preserved left ventricular systolic dysfunction) from the late 1960s (Wood), the early 1990s (Packer) and the modern era (ESC – 2005 guidelines).

In most cases of *symptomatic* CHF (if one accepts the majority view that CHF has to involve a component of clinical symptoms that typically, but not always, respond to targeted therapy), the syndrome involves the combination of the following:
- Left ventricular dysfunction (systolic or diastolic).
- Abnormal neurohormonal regulation.

- Unmet metabolic demand.
- Breathlessness and intolerance to exercise.
- Fluid retention.
- Premature death.

In typically old and fragile individuals CHF is rarely an isolated condition. Comorbidities that form part of, or negatively interact with, the pathology summarized below commonly include renal and respiratory failure, anemia and, of course, other chronic manifestations of the disease [83].

Pathogenesis of chronic heart failure (adapted from Krum et al. [84])

Chronic heart failure occurs in the context of a diverse group of disorders that reduce or alter myocardial performance and subsequently leads to the syndrome described above. In general terms, ventricular impairment may result from any of the following:

- Conditions that directly impair regional or global cardiac muscle function (most commonly AMI or cardiomyopathy).
- Conditions that cause chronic pressure (most commonly aortic stenosis and chronic hypertension) or volume overload (most commonly mitral regurgitation) overload.
- Uncontrolled acute and chronic arrhythmias (most commonly AF).
- Diseases involving the pericardium (this is the rarest cause of CHF) [84].

In order to tailor therapy it is vitally important to comprehensively evaluate the underlying etiology and duration of ventricular dysfunction. In an attempt to categorize the pathophysiologic processes that contribute to the symptomatic basis for CHF, it is common for this syndrome to be considered in terms of the following:

- Left ventricular systolic dysfunction (e.g. a left ventricular ejection fraction of $\leq 45\%$), or, in the presence of apparently "preserved" systolic function (such dysfunction may be demonstrated on exercise only).
- Abnormalities of diastolic performance (so-called "diastolic heart failure") [84].

It is quite probable that emerging advances in ultrasound techniques (including tissue Doppler and strain imaging) are likely to improve our understanding of myocardial properties in systolic and diastolic heart failure. However, Figure 1.9 shows the dramatic difference (on postmortem) between a heart that failed due to an acute ischemic insult and regionally impaired systolic dysfunction (left panel) and a grossly enlarged heart that also failed whilst maintaining "adequate" systolic function (right panel) as determined by left ventricular ejection fraction.

Systolic dysfunction

At a global level, the failing ventricle is characterized by ventricular dilatation and hypertrophy with an associated increase in wall stress (see left panel of Figure 1.9). This process is initially associated with maintained resting cardiac

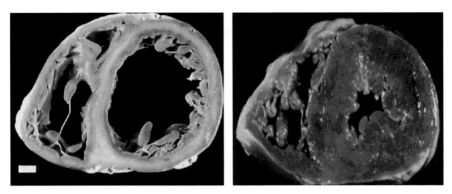

Figure 1.9 Post-mortem characteristics of systolic (right panel) versus diastolic dysfunction (left panel).

output, although the cardiac output response to exercise is diminished [84]. At the cellular level milder forms of systolic failure are reflected initially in an inability to recruit contractile function during stress (such as in response to catecholamines or increased rate). Only at the end-stage does "basal" myocyte contractility fail substantively. A number of key mechanisms contribute to loss of myocyte contractile function:

1 Alterations in intracellular calcium homeostasis which result from changes in the expression and activity of key proteins including the sarcoplasmic reticulum Ca^{2+} ATPase and phospholamban [85].
2 Alterations in the expression and function of adrenergic receptors [86].
3 Changes in the expression and function of contractile proteins themselves [87].
4 Activation of processes that lead to programmed death of myocytes (apoptosis) [87].

In the course of progressive heart failure it is well recognized that the ventricle dilates and assumes a more spherical geometry ("remodeling"). Left ventricular dilatation results in changes in the ventricular geometry and may also be associated with the development of secondary mitral regurgitation due to malformation and pressure on the mitral valve. These morphological changes are also often accompanied by a component of myocardial fibrosis which adversely impacts on diastolic chamber stiffness [84].

Diastolic dysfunction

It is now evident that abnormal diastolic function accompanies nearly all forms of CHF. In this context, it is important to note that diastolic function is particularly sensitive to ischemia. Any alterations in diastolic performance are likely to reflect underlying alterations in ventricular stiffness: myocardial fibrosis due to collagen deposition has been proposed as a key determinant of ventricular stiffness in the setting of CHF. In assessing "diastolic" function on

the basis of the active and passive elements of ventricular diastole, it is also relevant to take into account the influence of the following factors:
- Volume overload.
- The interaction of the left and right ventricle (via the interventricular septum).
- The constraining effect of the pericardium on an enlarged heart [84].

Ultimately all of these factors will combine to influence the ventricular end diastolic pressure, a key determinant of symptomatic status.

Neurohormonal activation

In CHF the underlying problem of decreased cardiac output activates many neurohormonal compensatory systems that, in the short term, act to *preserve* circulatory homeostasis and maintain arterial pressure [88]. However, when chronically activated, these compensatory systems play a key role in the development and progression of the syndrome. Early compensatory mechanisms include activation of the sympathetic nervous system and the renin-angiotensin system, leading to elevated levels of noradrenaline, angiotensin II and aldosterone and, more latterly, elevated levels of vasopressin and endothelin [88,89]. These mediators actively work against optimal cardiac function via increased peripheral resistance and adverse effects on cardiac structure, causing hypertrophy and fibrosis, myocyte necrosis and/or apoptosis, as well as downregulation of beta-adrenergic receptors and endothelial dysfunction [88,89]. In the early stages of CHF, the adverse effects of endogenous vasoconstrictors are balanced by elevated levels of the natriuretic peptides, which cause vasodilation and also inhibit the secretion of noradrenaline, renin, and vasopressin. In advanced CHF, the actions of vasodilator systems are attenuated, resulting in unopposed vasoconstrictor systems and consequent systemic and pulmonary vasoconstriction, cardiac hypertrophy and ischemia, edema, and hyponatremia [84]. The clinical importance of activation of neurohormones in CHF is two-fold:
- Circulating levels reflect LV function and predict prognosis.
- Blockade of the actions of angiotensin and noradrenaline slows progression of myocardial dysfunction, alleviates symptoms and reduces morbidity and mortality [84].

The various processes described above and that lead to progressive CHF (and ultimately death) are summarized in Figure 1.10.

Other key pathological processes in CHF

In addition to the key pathological changes in cardiac and neuroendocrine function outlined above, there are number of other key processes that contribute to the syndrome. For example, major alterations in regional blood flow have been consistently observed in CHF: these changes largely reflect the combined influences of increased vasoconstrictor system activity and reduced activity of endothelium-dependent vasodilatory processes, most notably the nitric oxide pathway. Structural changes, including vascular wall edema and

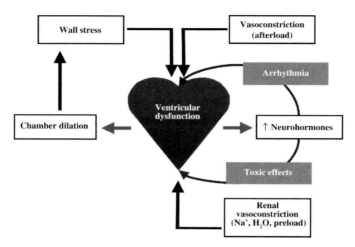

Figure 1.10 Pathogenesis of chronic heart failure.

reduced vascular density, may also occur and lead to progressive CHF. More-over, it is now accepted that there are key changes in muscle metabolism that could contribute to exercise intolerance [84]. These changes are independent of blood flow and are probably caused by a reduction in the mitochondrial content of skeletal muscle: importantly, exercise training ameliorates these metabolic changes [84]. Cardiac cachexia, sometimes a prominent feature of severe CHF, includes loss of muscle mass as well as adipose tissue. Cardiac cachexia may be caused by increased production of tumor necrosis factor; particularly in severe CHF [90,91].

Pathophysiologic consequences of chronic heart failure

The inevitable consequences of the processes described above are best en-capsulated by Figure 1.11 (adapted from original report) showing the typical decline in clinical status of individuals with CHF that is characterized by recur-rent episodes of clinical instability and an inevitable death. Two large studies from the USA have shown that CHF impairs self-reported quality of life more than any other common chronic medical disorder [92,93]. These findings have been confirmed by a more contemporary European study [94]. Not surpris-ingly, quality of life deteriorates with increasing heart failure severity, and this is associated with increased numbers of physician visits, drug consumption, and hospitalization. The prevalence of major depression in older patients hos-pitalized with CHF is particularly high (more than one third of individuals are typically affected) [95]. Such depression is both prolonged and largely un-treated in patients with chronic heart failure [96,97]. Dyspnea, confusion and pain are also very common during the last few days of life in heart failure. The majority of patients would prefer "comfort care" and do not wish active resuscitation. Many would even prefer death [98,99].

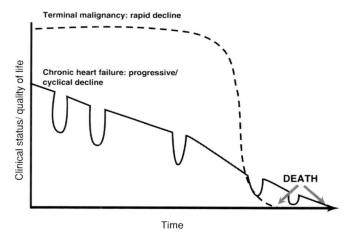

Figure 1.11 The typical trajectory of clinical and functional decline in chronic heart failure (Adapted from Lynn, 1997, [109]).

As will be noted repeatedly throughout this book, chronic cardiac disease (and CHF in particular) is commonly associated with recurrent hospitalization. In the USA, like many other countries, CHF has been identified as the most common cause of hospitalization in people over the age of 65 years [100]. An admission for CHF is frequently prolonged and in many cases followed by readmission within a short period of time [101]. Within the UK about one-third of patients are readmitted within 12 months of discharge [102], whilst the same proportion are reported to readmitted within six months in the USA [100,101]. Such readmission rates are usually higher than the other major causes of hospitalization, including stroke, hip fracture and respiratory disease [101]. On a sex-specific basis, men tend to be younger than women when admitted for the first time with CHF, but because of greater female longevity, the number of male and female admissions is roughly equal. Moreover the average age of individuals experiencing their first admission for CHF appears to be increasing [102,103].

In addition to being remarkably debilitating, CHF is a truly "malignant" condition. For example, in the original and subsequent Framingham cohorts, the probability of someone dying within five years of being diagnosed with heart failure was between 62% and 75% in men and 38% and 42% in women respectively. In comparison, five-year survival for all cancers among men and women in the USA during the same period was approximately 50% [103]. A range of studies from the UK, USA, and Canada has specifically addressed this issue [104–109]. It was within this context that we recently compared five-year survival rates for all Scottish patients admitted for the first time with CHF in 1991 with those Scottish patients admitted for the first time with the most common types of cancer (specific to men and women) in addition to

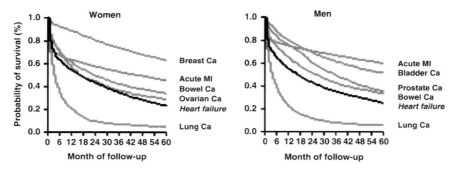

Figure 1.12 Five-year survival rates for all Scottish patients with CHF compared to most common types of cancer (specific to men and women) in addition to acute myocardial infarction [105].

acute myocardial infarction [105]. Figure 1.12 [105] shows the crude, five-year survival rates for each diagnosis. Multivariate analysis showed that, with the major exception of lung cancer, CHF was associated with the poorest longer-term, adjusted survival in men.

In women both cancer of the breast and large bowel were associated with better short-term survival rates in comparison to CHF. Consistent with more recent data from the Framingham Study [107], it was found that CHF was associated with a significant number of "premature" life-years lost (on average nine years per person), being associated with more deaths than the combination of large bowel, prostate and bladder cancer. In women, despite the fact that proportionately more deaths occurred in those who had already exceeded average life expectancy, CHF was second only to AMI in terms of the total number of premature deaths. Both lung and breast cancer, however, by virtue of a greater number of expected life-years lost per person had a greater impact on the population as a whole during this period [105]. Approximately half of all deaths in those unfortunate to develop CHF are sudden (hence the emergence of automated internal defibrillators [110]), the remaining portion being typically associated with progressive cardiorespiratory and/or renal dysfunction. Although there is evidence from population studies that survival rates are improving [103,111] with the introduction of new and more effective therapies that slow progression of the complex processes outlined above (see the next chapter for treatment options) there is still no *cure* for CHF.

Defining and classifying chronic atrial fibrillation

Atrial fibrillation is a supraventricular tachyarrhythmia caused by disorganized and rapid atrial depolarizations without effective atrial contraction. As shown in the rhythm strip below (Figure 1.13), electrocardiography reveals small baseline irregularities of variable amplitude and morphology (fibrillation waves). Although the atrial rate is typically between 300 and 600 beats per minute, the ventricular rate is usually between 100 and 150 beats per

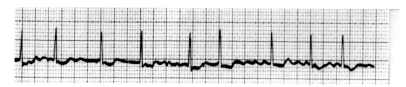

Figure 1.13 Atrial fibrillation on an ECG rhythm strip.

minute and irregular. As such, a normally functioning atrioventricular (AV) node, with its relatively high depolarization threshold, is essential to "buffering" the ventricles from completely mirroring the fast, ineffectual beats of the atria.

Atrial fibrillation may occur in isolation in up to 10% of cases (so-called "lone" AF when an individual is aged <65 years [112]) but, significantly in the context of this book, most commonly occurs in the presence of underlying cardiovascular disease. Contemporary ACC/AHA/ESC Guidelines have classified AF on the following basis [113]:

- First detected.
- Paroxysmal AF that is self-terminating: the majority of episodes are of less than 24 hours duration but can last for up to seven days and may be recurrent in nature.
- Persistent AF that is not self-terminating and may require treatment in the form of chemical or electrical cardioversion (so called "rhythm control" management): left untreated, episodes may last longer than seven days and may be recurrent in nature.
- Permanent AF: may take the form of paroxysmal or persistent AF, however, either due to a clinical decision to limit the underlying ventricular rate (so-called "rate control" management) or due to failed cardioversion, patients require chronic treatment [113].

Pathogenesis of atrial fibrillation

Persistent and permanent AF is the most common form of this arrhythmia and is responsible for the largest proportion of morbid and fatal events described below. As such, there are a number of underlying disease states that both increase the likelihood of an individual developing paroxysmal and persistent AF – particularly when a triggering event occurs. Some of the major "triggers" of AF include [113]:

- Excessive alcohol intake (so-called "holiday heart").
- Cardiothoracic surgery.
- Electrocution.
- Acute myocardial ischemia.
- Pericarditis/myocarditis.
- Pulmonary diseases.
- Hyperthyroidism and other metabolic disease states [113].

Clearly, there are a number "triggers" particularly relevant to the individual with another form of chronic cardiac disease (e.g. heart failure and chronic angina pectoris). Atrial fibrillation may also be triggered by excess parasympathetic or sympathetic tone (e.g. vagal AF [114]). The latter has been postulated as a major reason for increased AF-morbidity and mortality in winter months. [115,116]. Not surprisingly, underlying heart disease is considered to be the major cause of AF; it is clear that advancing age with all its associated changes in the structural and mechanical efficiencies of the heart increases the likelihood of developing AF. In Framingham cohorts the following were all independently associated with an increased risk of developing AF in the longer-term [117]:

- Each decade of incremental age = 2.1-fold and 2.2-fold increased risk in men and women, respectively.
- Diabetes = 1.4 and 1.6-fold increased risk.
- Underlying hypertension = 1.5 and 1.4-fold increased risk.
- Congestive heart failure = 4.5 and 5.9-fold increased risk.
- Valvular heart disease (usually affecting the mitral valve) = 1.8 and 3.4-fold increased risk.
- Past AMI = 1.4-fold increased risk in men only [117].

In terms of population attributable risk the risk factors most important in terms of potentially preventing new cases of AF were hypertension (14%) and CHF (10%). In women the most important risk factors in this regard were valvular disease (18%), hypertension (14%), CHF (12%), and cigarette smoking (8%) [118].

Patients with persistent AF often display structural abnormalities, other than left atrial enlargement, that cannot be completely explained by underlying heart disease [119]. Fibrosis and inflammation are two processes that are commonly identified with such changes: although determining which comes first (i.e. before or after the development of AF) is problematic. Two predominant pathophysiologic processes have been described in relation to AF:

1 Enhanced automaticity in one or more rapidly depolarizing foci – typically in the superior pulmonary veins.

2 Reentry involving one or more circuits (multiple wavelet hypothesis) [120].

It is important to note that AF, unlike those arrhythmias typically affecting the ventricles, probably involves multiple reentrant circuits and there is some evidence to suggest that it involves sequential wave fronts occurring at regular intervals [121]. However, there is much more to be understood about the pathophysiology of AF in all its forms.

It has been long known that "AF begets AF", in that the longer it has persisted the harder it is to treat with particularly high rates of resistance to electrical or chemical cardioversion as well as high rates of recurrence even if successful cardioversion is initially achieved. Both rates are particularly high when "real life" cohorts are examined. [122] Such "resistance" has been linked to the phenomenon of "electrophysiological remodelling" where repeated bursts of initially paroxysmal AF are associated with progressive shortening of effective refractory periods and increasing episode duration. [123,124]. There is recent evidence to suggest that decreased inward current through L-type calcium channels plays an important role in this process [125]. Furthermore, persistent AF adversely affects atrial contractile function and sinus node recovery time and may contribute to the common phenomenon of sick sinus syndrome characterized by alternating episodes of tachycardia and bradycardia common to many older patients with chronic heart disease [126].

The loss of the "atrial kick" to ventricular filling and the loss of synchronous activity within the heart as a whole in AF will have an immediate and deleterious hemodynamic effect – particularly in the setting of CHF. It is important to note that a persistently high ventricular rate in the presence of AF has also been shown to induce a tachycardia-induced cardiomyopathy affecting both the atria and ventricles and resulting in consequent CHF [127]. Overall, however, thrombus formation in the left atrium leading to ischemic stroke [128] is undoubtedly, the most recognized consequence of persistent AF. The risk of stroke is as high as 5% per annum in those aged 75 years or more without prophylactic treatment for underlying AF [129]. A number of studies have confirmed that AF itself confers a hypercoagulable state in affected individuals. As such, a hypercoagulable state in AF is also additive to the presence of structural and flow abnormalities that fulfill Virchow's triad for thrombus formation [130,131]. Clinically important and measurable predictors of spontaneous echo contrast indicative of emboli in the left atrium, include left atrial size, left atrial appendage flow velocity, underlying left ventricular dysfunction, fibrinogen levels, hematocrit and presence of aortic atherosclerosis [113].

Pathophysiologic consequences of atrial fibrillation

As a truly "malignant" arrhythmia, AF contributes to a significant and increasing component of cardiovascular-related morbidity in developed countries (see next section). During a 38-year follow-up of the Framingham Heart Cohort in the US, AF was associated with an adjusted 1.5–1.9-fold increased risk of death in men and women [118]. Similarly, during 20-year follow-up of the Renfrew-Paisley cohort in the UK, AF was associated with a 1.5–2.2-fold increased risk of all cause death and a 1.8–2.8-fold increased risk of a cardiovascular-related death in men and women, respectively [130]. Not unexpectedly, a major cause of premature death in those with AF is ischemic stroke. In the Framingham Heart Study, AF was associated with a 4–5-fold increased risk of stroke, its prognostic importance becoming more acute in this regard with advanced age [127]. For example, the population attributable risk of AF-related stroke mortality increased from 1.5% in those aged 50–59 years to 24% in those aged 80–89 years [127]. As noted above, it is becoming increasingly more evident that persistent AF also confers an increased risk of developing CHF. Together with stroke, CHF is the most debilitating and deadly of cardiovascular disease states [131]. In the Renfrew/Paisley cohort, AF detected in middle-age was associated with a 3.4-fold increased risk of developing CHF in both men and women [130]. Regardless of the exact relationship between AF and CHF, the two are often found in the same patient. For example, in Scotland the proportion of <u>all</u> patients hospitalized with a diagnosis of AF and a concurrent coding of CHF was approximately 15% in 1996 [132]. In a more contemporary report from Denmark, the equivalent figure in 1999 was 24% [133].

1.4 Epidemiologic burden of the most common manifestations of chronic cardiac disease

Chronic angina pectoris

A recent study examined the burden imposed by the most common symptomatic manifestation of CAD, angina pectoris, on the National Health Service in the United Kingdom in the year 2000 [134]. The United Kingdom (population 60 million) has a universal health care system and detailed utilization and expenditure data that enables a more detailed analysis of these parameters when compared to other countries with more "fractionated" health care systems. Using the best available data, the study conservatively estimated that during the year 2000 angina pectoris consumed more than 1% of health care expenditure. More specifically, it estimated that during the year 2000:

- 634,000 patients (1.1% of the total population) being actively managed for angina pectoris by their local primary care physician.
- These patients required 2.4 million primary care visits for their condition.
- There were one quarter of a million referrals to hospital outpatient clinics for specialist investigation and management.
- There were 16 million prescriptions to treat angina pectoris (predominantly nitrates).
- The total cost of community management of angina pectoris was £172 million (the equivalent of almost three pounds sterling per person).
- There were almost 150,000 admissions for angina/unstable angina (i.e. not including acute myocardial infarction).
- There were almost 120,000 coronary angiograms, coronary artery bypass-grafts and percutaneous coronary angioplasty procedures with or without a coronary stent.
- Hospitalized patients required more than half a million outpatient visits (not including cardiac rehabilitation).
- The total cost of hospital-based management of angina pectoris was almost £500 million (the equivalent of more than eight pounds sterling per person) [134].

Figure 1.14 summarizes the overall burden imposed by angina pectoris in the UK during the year 2000. The British Heart Foundation also estimates that the total number of people with a history of angina (i.e. not necessarily treated but still contributing to disability levels) in 2000/2001 was 2 million (3.3% of the total population). There were also an additional 275,000 myocardial infarctions in that year that would have conservatively cost an additional £1.5 billion (an additional 4% of National Health Service expenditure) [135].

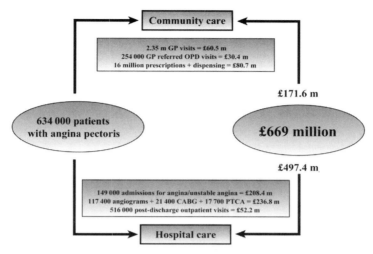

Figure 1.14 Summary of the economic burden of angina pectoris in the United Kingdom in the year 2000 [134].

Overall, it has been estimated that coronary heart disease costs £7.5 billion in direct and indirect expenditure in that country [135]. In the United States it is now estimated that heart disease costs $US 142.1 billion (2005 figure) per annum. In 1999 alone, Medicare beneficiaries were paid $US 11 billion and the number of coronary angiograms (predominantly triggered by angina pectoris) has risen exponentially, along with other invasive procedures in the past two decades (from 300,000 in 1979 to 1.4 million in 2002) [136].

Chronic heart failure

An increasing number of population studies have quantified the number of individuals affected by CHF using different criteria (see Figure 1.14). In recognition of the inherent limitations of defining CHF on the basis of clinical signs and symptoms in the absence of determining the presence or absence of underlying structural or functional heart disease and further recognition that heart failure is not necessarily confined to those with impaired systolic dysfunction but can arise when systolic function appears to be *preserved* (so-called diastolic heart failure), an increasing number of epidemiologic studies that have directly measured cardiac function have been undertaken. Those studies that included more than 1000 subjected and some form of objective measure are summarized in Table 1.4. In most cases these studies have estimated left ventricular ejection fraction via echocardiography. Based on such data we now know that in the geographic regions of Europe (6.5 million), Japan (2.4 million), the USA (5 million) and Australia (0.4 million) a combined total of almost 15 million people are directly affected by CHF [137].

Table 1.4 Proportion of people with symptomatic or asymptomatic left ventricular systolic dysfunction, or normal/preserved left ventricular systolic function in epidemiological studies of heart failure [138–146].

Location	Subjects	Ages	Mean age	Definition of LVSD	LVSD (%)	Symptom-free (%)
Glasgow (Scotland) [138]	1640	25–74	50	LVEF ≤ 30%	2.9	48
				LVEF ≤ 35%	7.7	77
Birmingham (England) [139]	3960	> 45	61	LVEF < 40%	1.8	47
				LVEF < 50%	5.3	61
Rotterdam (The Netherlands) [140]	1698	55–95	65	FS ≤ 25%	3.7	60
Augsburg (Germany) [141]	1866	25–75	50	LVEF < 48%	2.7	42
Various-CHS (USA) [142]	5201	65–100	73	Abnormal*	3.7	
Various-SHS (USA) [143]	3184	45–74	60	Mild (LVEF 40–54%)	11.1	95[†]
				Severe (LVEF < 40%)	2.9	72[†]
Copenhagen (Denmark) [144]	2158	≥ 50		FS < 0.26	2.9	34

Location	Subjects	Ages	Mean age	Prevalence of CHF (%)	Preserved systolic function (%)
Various-CHS (USA) [145]	4842	66–103	78	8.8	55
Rotterdam (The Netherlands) [140]	1698	55–95	65	2.1	71
Various-SHS (USA) [142]	3184	47–81	60	3.0	53
Portugal [146]	5434	> 25	68	4.4	39

LVSD = Left ventricular systolic dysfunction; CHS = Cardiovascular Health Study; FS = fractional shortening of the left ventricle; LVEF = left ventricular ejection fraction; SHS = Strong Heart Study (American Indians).
*Qualitative/semiquantitative assessment of left ventricular systolic function.
[†] No heart failure.

Some of the most reliable epidemiological data on CHF come from reports of hospital admissions on a country-by-country basis: although these need to be interpreted with some caution owing to their retrospective nature, variations in coding practices, and changing admission thresholds over time. It is important to note that reports from diverse countries such as Scotland [147], Spain [148], the USA [149], Sweden [150], New Zealand [151], and The Netherlands [152] relating to the period 1978 to 1994 showed that heart failure-related admission rates were increasing. For example, studies undertaken in the UK suggest that 0.2% of the population in the early 1990s were hospitalized for heart failure per annum, and that such admissions accounted for more than 5% of adult general medicine and geriatric hospital admissions – outnumbering those associated with AMI [147]. In the USA CHF is the most common cause of hospitalization in people over the age of 65 years [49,100].

Preliminary reports from Scotland [153] and The Netherlands [154], now supported by similar data from Singapore [155] and Sweden [156] suggest that the population rate of admissions associated with a primary diagnosis of CHF have begun to plateau. However, there is little doubt that age-adjusted admission rates in older individuals continue to rise and the absolute number of admissions, as a reflection of older societies overall, will also rise. Overall, the duration of hospital stay associated with CHF is frequently prolonged and in many cases is rapidly followed by readmission. Within the UK about one-third of patients are readmitted within 12 months of discharge [153], whilst the same proportion are reported to be readmitted within six months in the USA [157]. Such readmission rates are usually higher than the other major causes of hospitalization, including stroke, hip fracture, and respiratory disease [157]. A recent comparison of readmission rates associated with a number of conditions in three States in the USA and three European countries has highlighted the difficulty in comparing different regions due to confounding variables [157]. However, as expected, CHF, along with chronic pulmonary disease was associated with the highest readmission rates in both the US and Europe [157].

In the 1990s it was estimated that the overall cost of managing CHF consumed a significant amount (1–2%) of health-care expenditure in developed countries [158]. Not surprisingly, hospitalizations represent the costliest (more than two thirds) component of such expenditure [158]. Given the likelihood of an increasing number (if not population rates) of heart failure-related hospitalizations in these countries, it is likely that these reported estimates fall short of the current burden it imposes. Data from the UK best illustrates the increasing cost of CHF in developed countries (see Figure 1.15) [158].

In 1990 CHF was estimated to cost 1.3% of health care expenditure [158]. Based on a more contemporary estimate, for the year 2000 it is now estimated to consume approximately 2.1% of expenditure (based on 1990 equivalent expenditure levels) and, when the cost of hospitalization associated with a secondary diagnosis of CHF is also considered, this figure rises markedly to 4% [159]. The comparative profile of CHF in the UK for the year 2000, relative to that shown for angina pectoris (see Figure 4.1) (the same methods were used to derive key estimates) is presented in Figure 1.16 [159].

Given the complicated messages imparted by indications that the common precursors of CHF are under some control but some new precursors (e.g. obesity [160]) are not, trends indicating falling incidence rates and what appears to be more prolonged survival associated with the syndrome, predicting the future is fraught with uncertainty. However, the progressive ageing of the population (i.e. substantially more people at risk of developing heart disease, hypertension and then CHF) is a known factor that is likely to require a major

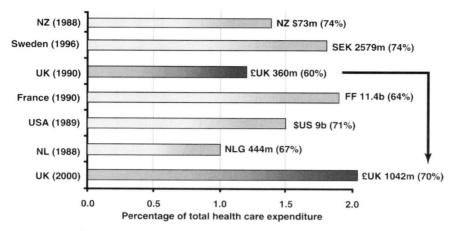

Figure 1.15 The increasing cost of chronic heart failure in developed countries [158]. Percentages shown in parentheses represent the proportion of expenditure relating to hospital-based costs (FF, French francs; NLG, Netherlands guilders; SEK, Swedish kronor; b, billion; m, million).

change in the underlying incidence of CHF to prevent a sustained epidemic. Based on recent trends demonstrating that the related epidemic has indeed stabilized but will likely be magnified by the ageing of the population, we recently reported the likely impact of current trends on the prevalence and morbidity associated with CHF in Scotland – see Figure 1.17 [161]. This figure shows that the most likely scenario is a gradual but still substantial increase in CHF-related prevalence and health care activity over the next decade and

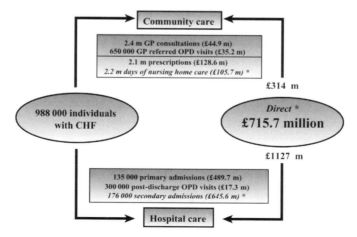

Figure 1.16 Comparative profile of chronic heart failure in the UK for the year 2000, relative to that shown for angina pectoris [159].

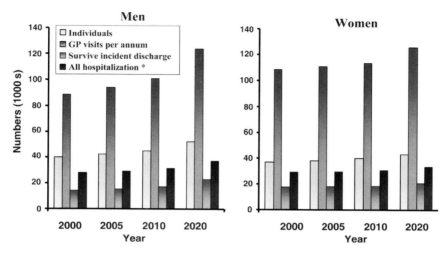

Figure 1.17 The likely impact of current trends on the prevalence and morbidity associated with CHF in Scotland over the next 15 years [161].

beyond. Overall, it is projected that the number of men and women affected by CHF will increase by 31% and 17% respectively, with 52% more male and 16% more female incident admissions, respectively [161]. Certainly, these figures are far less dramatic than previously predicted [162,163] and the prediction that more men than women affected is markedly different from the current profile of CHF in many countries.

There is little doubt, therefore, that the doubling in CHF-related costs in the UK during the period 1990–2000 will not be an isolated event – particularly given the prediction of increasing CHF-related hospitalizations. As the experience of CHF has been remarkably similar in all developed countries there is also little doubt that its "international" cost will also continue to rise without substantial changes in its prevention and management.

Chronic atrial fibrillation

Using large-scale, population-based data, Feinberg and colleagues estimated that 0.9% of the US population (2.2 million) in 1995 was affected by paroxysmal or sustained AF at any one time [164]. Similarly, using reliable UK data, it was estimated that a similar proportion of the UK population were affected by AF that year [165]. Based on the ageing UK population and increasing prevalence rates, it was further estimated that the prevalence of AF had risen to just over 1% of the UK population in the year 2000 [165]. Large population-based studies [117,130,165,166] show a clear linear relationship between the prevalence of AF and advancing age: in developed countries, more than 5% of those aged 65 years or more are likely to be affected by AF at any one time and, as shown above, the proportion of such individuals within the population is steadily increasing.

Regardless of the cohort and type of study, AF has been shown to be a significant marker of future morbidity. For example, a small number of epidemiologic studies have examined the rate of AF-related hospitalization over a prolonged period of follow-up in specific population cohorts. For example, Wilhelmen and colleagues examined incident admissions relating to AF in the Multifactor Primary Prevention Study cohort in Sweden. During 27 years follow-up (mean 25.2 years), a total of 754 men (10.1%) were hospitalized with AF as a principal or contributory diagnosis [167]. Similarly, we examined the frequency of AF-related admissions in the similarly aged Renfrew/Paisley cohort in the UK over a shorter period (i.e. they were younger at the completion of study follow-up). During a 20-year follow-up, a similar proportion of men and women (3.6% and 3.4%, respectively) were discharged from hospital with a diagnosis of AF [166].

A number of studies have now examined trends in hospitalizations associated with AF in whole populations. In a study of the number of patients discharged from short-stay hospitals in the USA between 1982 and 1993 with a diagnosis of AF, a 2.1-fold increase in such admissions was observed [168]. This increase was observed in both the elderly (from 30.6 to 59.5/10,000 in those aged $\geq$65 years) and younger patients (from 7.9 to 11.5/10,000 in those aged $\leq$65 years) [168]. Similar increases have been observed in Scotland during the period 1985–1996. For example, the population rate of AF-related admissions in men rose from 7.3 to 16.6/10,000 in those aged 45–65 years and from 16.6 to 54.9/10,000 in those aged $\geq$65 years [169]. Figure 1.18 shows the dramatic increase in the total number of AF-related admissions observed during this period in Scotland. In a recent examination of incident admissions for AF in

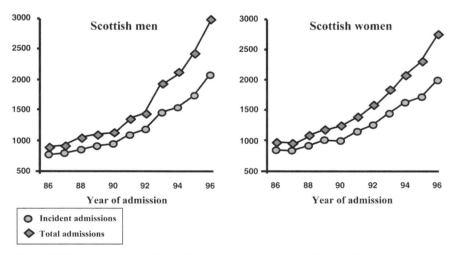

Figure 1.18 Total number of AF-related admissions observed in Scotland during the period of 1985–1996 [169].

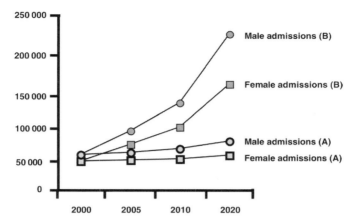

Figure 1.19 Predicted future burden of atrial fibrillation in the UK [171].

Denmark during the period 1980–1990, Frost and colleagues found that the annual incidence of AF increased from 1.98/10,000 individuals aged 40–89 years in 1980 to 4.38/10,000 individual in the same age group in 1999 [133].

Given that the population prevalence of AF has increased dramatically in the past two decades, it is more than likely to continue rise in the foreseeable future because of two interrelating factors that have already underpinned the well documented epidemic of CHF described above [170]. Firstly, improved survival rates in those with coronary heart disease and hypertension (two common precursors of AF) and, secondly, the general ageing of the population. Based on the Scottish data described above, it has been calculated that the number of men and women being treated for AF in the UK will increase from about 550,000 (just under 1% of the total population) to 800,000 by the year 2020 [171]. This represents a 45% increase in cases of AF over two decades. Similar rises have been predicted in the US population [164,168]. Figure 1.19 shows the likely increase in AF-related hospitalization (primary diagnosis only) in Scotland based on population changes alone (Model A) or, the more likely scenario, of steadily increasing hospitalization rates combined with the ageing population (Model B): the latter profile is similar to that observed in relation to CHF during the last two decades of the 20th century [167]. Given that there is no cure for coronary heart disease, only better palliative treatment, and the progressive ageing of the population, most experts agree that the epidemic of AF is likely to be sustained in the foreseeable future.

The likely rise in AF-related hospitalization rates is extremely significant given that like many other chronic disease states (particularly CHF), AF exerts is greatest cost burden on the hospital sector (see section above). However, there have been very few studies that have specifically quantified the economic burden of AF in the same way that other significant cardiac disease states such as stroke [172] and CHF [159]. As AF is a major trigger for stroke,

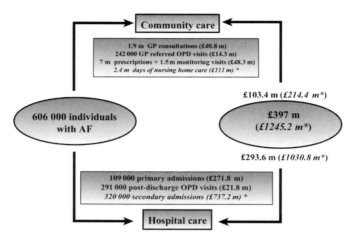

Figure 1.20 Summary of the economic burden of atrial fibrillation in the United Kingdom (year 2000) [165].

chronic heart failure, respiratory failure and a major complication following open- heart surgery, it undoubtedly exerts a significant burden on the health care system but is largely underestimated [165]. For example, a recent study of resource utilization related to AF following coronary artery bypass grafting in the US, found that 33% of patients developed AF postoperatively for the first time and that they had significantly higher post-operative charges (mean difference $US 6356: $P < 0.001$) compared to those without AF [173]. Using the same methodology as that used to calculate the cost of angina pectoris [134] and CHF [159] we recently examined the cost of AF to the National Health Service in the UK during the years 1995 and 2000 [165]. During this period we estimated that the direct cost of AF had increased by over 50% [165]. As such it currently consumes around 1% of health care expenditure and indirectly contributes to an additional 2% of such costs [165]. As expected, hospital admissions account for about 60% of AF-related expenditure [165]. It should be noted once again, however, that the majority of health care activity relating to AF and other forms of chronic cardiac disease, occurs in the community. As indicated by Figure 1.20 major health care costs include visits to general practitioners and drug therapy – particularly anticoagulation therapy requiring active monitoring of coagulation status [165].

1.5 The overall cost burden of chronic cardiac disease

In order to place these three common manifestations of chronic cardiac disease into perspective, Figure 1.21 shows their relative cost to the UK health care system in the year 2000 [134,159,165]. It should be noted that the cost of these chronic conditions is not duplicated and that while they consumed

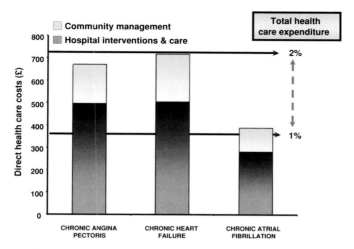

Figure 1.21 Relative cost to UK health system in the year 2000 of three most common chronic cardiac diseases: chronic angina pectoris, chronic heart failure, and chronic atrial fibrillation [134,159,165].

a combined 5% of direct health care expenditure in that country, when considering their interaction with other cardiovascular conditions (e.g. stroke) this cost rises to more than 10% of health care expenditure. Moreover, given that UK revascularization procedures are far below those commonly applied in the United States and Europe [174], sensitivity analyses showed that these expensive procedures would increase the cost of angina pectoris by more than 15% and that cardiac rehabilitation most probably cost an additional 11% in health care expenditure for that condition [134]. Similarly, when considering the emergence of CHF management programs [175] and invasive devices (e.g. implantable cardiac defibrillators and sophisticated pacing devices) the likely cost of managing CHF will continue to rise dramatically in the foreseeable future without dramatic changes in the pattern of health care delivery (hence this book!!).

CHAPTER 2

Key therapeutic targets in chronic cardiac care

2.1 Introduction

As described in Chapter 1, the number of elderly individuals developing a chronic cardiac condition (whether it be chronic angina pectoris, CHF or AF), is likely to increase within ageing Western populations. Figure 2.1 outlines the typical case history of a male who had a number of strong risk factors for coronary heart disease in middle age, who eventually experienced a nonfatal acute coronary event (an inferior AMI) that, when combined with a long history of uncontrolled systolic hypertension, ultimately led to CHF, chronic angina pectoris (with a strong decubitus component due to cardiomyopathy), AF and sudden cardiac death. The complexities of managing such an individual with concurrent disease states that complicate the intention and application of treatment cannot be overstated. For example, many patients who would otherwise benefit from the prescription of an angiotensin receptor antagonist or a beta-blocker for CHF secondary to impaired left ventricular systolic dysfunction are unable to tolerate such therapy due to concurrent renovascular disease and/or sick sinus syndrome.

In effectively dealing with chronic cardiac disease, therefore, there are competing priorities that often complicate attempts to draw up clear and precise therapeutic goals from both the patient and treating health care professional's perspective [176]. As indicated by Figure 2.1, however, there are often clear phases in the natural history of chronic cardiac disease that "anchor" the mindset and purpose of supportive and therapeutic management of the underlying disease relative to an individual's life-situation (i.e. middle-age versus beyond normal life-expectancy). These phases include:

- *Primary prevention*. In the absence of any signs of overt symptoms of heart disease there is an onus on someone "at risk" (remembering that any ageing adult man or woman is at risk!) to adopt a healthy lifestyle to prevent its development – particularly sudden cardiac death. Supportive strategies at the primary care level to detect any underlying risk factors (e.g. obesity, Type II diabetes and/or hypertension) and address them via lifestyle advice (e.g. low-fat diet and greater exercise) and/or more active interventions (e.g. lipid-lowering agents) is essential to prevent or even delay the onset of heart disease. Of course, those who see little reason to seek treatment/advice

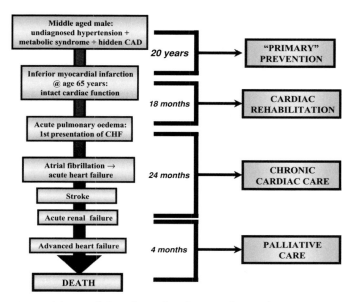

Figure 2.1 A case history of chronic cardiac disease: phases of management.

and/or adopt healthier lifestyles are clearly more likely to develop heart disease and move to the next phase!

- *Secondary prevention/cardiac rehabilitation.* Once an individual has "revealed" that they have underlying heart disease (most commonly due to a nonfatal syncopal attack, cardiac arrest or acute coronary syndrome), the health care system moves into "high alert" to prevent the survivors from rapidly progressing towards a chronic or even rapidly terminal cardiac condition: sometimes this is unavoidable, but, as noted in Chapter 1, there is evidence to suggest that we are becoming more adept, at the population level, at delaying the onset of chronic cardiac disease (most notably CHF). Secondary prevention often occurs in isolation to primary prevention, in that many individuals do not represent "primary prevention failures" but are new to the preventative process: even though it now occurs when they have developed an overt version of the disease. The key principles of modifying major risk factors, however, remain the same with the exception that affected individuals are typically symptom-free once they have received definitive treatment (e.g. undergoing placement of a drug-eluting stent for an occlusive lesion in the left-anterior descending coronary artery that triggered an acute coronary syndrome).
- *Chronic cardiac care.* It is only when an individual is chronically impaired or affected by ongoing symptoms relating to their underlying heart disease that the concept of chronic cardiac care is applied. Often this occurs when "secondary prevention" fails and they suffer a second or even third event (e.g. a

recurrent AMI). Unfortunately, there are very few studies that have examined the natural history of heart disease in a whole population. Anecdotal evidence suggests that the permutations for acute on chronic manifestations of heart disease are complex and that a generic and often "reactive" approach to management is often adopted. Clearly, this book outlines a more individualized and "proactive" approach to management by stressing the importance of maintaining "secondary prevention" and working with the individual and the best aspects of the local health care system in order to optimize treatment strategies (see Chapters 5 and 6) and improve subsequent health outcomes.

- *Palliative care*. Being proactive in terms of dealing with chronic cardiac disease at one end of the spectrum (i.e. when a person first requires careful management) also predicates being proactive at the other end of that disease spectrum: when the underlying heart disease has become terminal and irreversible and preventative and treatment strategies, therefore, have no relevance in terms of improving an individuals quality of life, but when the goal of ensuring a quality *end-of-life* becomes the primary objective of care. Viewed from a hierarchical perspective, it is pragmatic to consider the principles of management that underpin that phase of the patient's life cycle and cardiac pathology as "active" until clearly superseded by the competing priorities of the subsequent or even distal phase of the disease process (depending on the speed of transition and consolidation of cardiac function). As indicated by the title and articulated more fully in the Preface, this book is dedicated to improving outcomes in those who have already developed chronic cardiac disease. It is important to note, however, that rather than singularly focussing on "disease management" (refer to Chapter 4), this book strongly emphasizes the parallel need to address modifiable contributors (so-called risk factors) to the emergence of confounding and more disabling cardiovascular conditions (e.g. AF-related thromboembolic stroke), in addition to slowing the progression of the primary cardiac disease state (e.g. coronary artery disease) – (refer to Chapter 3). It also emphasizes the need to consider palliation (i.e. focussing on quality-end-of-life, instead of prolonging life through active interventions) when it is clear that an individual has reached the terminal phase of their disease process.

It is within this context that following sections of this chapter outline the key therapeutic goals that underpin the secondary prevention, treatment, and palliative care management of individuals affected by chronic cardiac disease. These sections are designed to provide an *overview* of the recommendations emanating from expert guidelines published via key organizations, (e.g. the European Society of Cardiology and the American Heart Association). As with other peak organizations dedicated to combating cardiovascular disease at the population level, both have specific processes for producing guidelines and, indeed, implementing them:

- "Get With The Guidelines[SM] (GWTG) is the premier hospital-based quality improvement program for the American Heart Association and the

American Stroke Association. It empowers health care provider teams to consistently treat patients with the most updated treatment guidelines." [http://www.americanheart.org/presenter.jhtml?identifier=1165–Accessed July 2005].

- "Essential documents for cardiology professionals and the related healthcare industry. ESC Guidelines are the flagship scientific products of the Society." [http://www.escardio.org/knowledge/guidelines/ – Accessed July 2005].

Most of the guidelines now produced by these organizations are available as "downloads" to personal computers and more practically, to handheld computers. However, it is important to reemphasize the need for a structured program to tailor individual management of patients in whom complex decisions need to be made based on the presence of parallel disease states, individual responses to treatment, and the overall context in which a person is living with, or indeed, dying from chronic cardiac disease.

2.2 Minimizing the impact of cardiac risk factors: a lifetime task

As indicated above, the arbitrary use of terms such as "primary" and "secondary" prevention mask the importance of minimizing the impact of modifiable risk factors not only before heart disease has occurred, but also after it has evolved into a chronic manifestation. The only time to stop any efforts to improve a person's risk-factor profile/susceptibility to disease progression, is when a conscious decision has been made to: (i) accept the full consequences of not addressing the "fuel(s)" that typically drive the progression of the disease (and therefore progressively debilitating symptoms) and/or, (ii) shift the focus of management to a predominantly palliative care approach.

The following therapeutic targets in relation to secondary prevention of heart disease are largely based on the following guidelines:

Smith SC Jr., Blair SN, Bonow RO, et al. on behalf of The Healthcare Professionals from the American Heart Association and the American College of Cardiology. AHA/ACC Guidelines for preventing heart attack and death in patients with atherosclerotic cardiovascular disease. 2001 update. *Circulation* 2001; **104**:1577–1579.

De Backer G, Ambrosioni E, Borch-Johnsen et al. on behalf of The Third Joint Task Force of the European and other societies on cardiovascular disease prevention in clinical practice. European guidelines on cardiovascular disease prevention in clinical practice. *Eur Heart J* 2003; **24**: 1601–1610.

Guiding principles of management. There is little doubt that there is increasing evidence to suggest that "aggressive" risk reduction on therapies for individuals with and without established cardiovascular disease have steadily reorientated the therapeutic targets (e.g. blood pressure and total cholesterol levels) that will yield the greatest benefits in terms of both "primary" and "secondary" prevention.

Key therapeutic targets. Table 2.1 is adapted from the summary statements issued by the AHA/ACC and ESC statements (listed above) in respect to the key therapeutic targets required to minimize the risk of further cardiovascular events in individuals already affected by the disease. These targets are a *constant* for all affected individuals unless treatment of the underlying process and/or complications from other conditions predicates otherwise. A conscious decision to "abandon" these targets should always be made on a proactive rather than passive basis.

Note: In primary prevention there are well-developed risk assessment tools (e.g. the ESCs Score System and the Framingham Cardiac Risk Assessment Score) to determine an individual's 5- to 10-year risk of experiencing a fatal cardiac event (typically taking into account their age, sex, smoking status, lipid profile, and blood pressure). It must be assumed that any individual who has survived an initial cardiac event and/or developed chronic symptoms is at high risk for a premature fatal event!

2.3 Living with cardiac disease: improving duration and quality of life

As discussed in Chapter 1, the most common manifestations of heart disease in our ageing populations, and the predominant focus of this book, are chronic angina pectoris, CHF, and AF. As such, they often represent the failure of both primary and secondary prevention strategies to completely halt the progressive nature of deteriorating cardiac function and structure due to the inevitable effects of age complicated by increased cardiac stress (e.g. due to systolic hypertension or valvular dysfunction) and/or repeated insults (e.g. due to myocardial ischemia).

Guiding principles. Although these three conditions typically emerge at different stages of the disease process and require distinct therapeutic strategies (see below) the overriding goals of management for these conditions are the same:
1 Slow and even reverse disease progression by addressing precipitating factors.
2 Minimize chronic disabling symptoms and therefore improve quality of life.
3 Minimize acute exacerbations that can impair quality of life and also lead to recurrently and costly hospitalizations and other expensive forms of health care.
4 Prolong survival without compromising on the quality of life.
As represented in Figure 2.1, these goals become progressively harder to achieve in those individuals who typically survive long enough to develop all three forms of chronic heart disease in addition to other significant forms

Table 2.1 Key therapeutic targets in secondary prevention.

Risk behavior/factor	Therapeutic target	Recommended action(s)
Smoking tobacco	Complete cessation	• Self-motivation to quit smoking • Supportive cessation programs • Avoid second-hand smoke • Nicotine replacement or buproprion
Hypertension	Minimum of $< 140/90$ mmHg OR $< 130/80$ in those with CHF, renal failure, or diabetes	• Lifestyle modification: weight control, exercise, moderate sodium intake, increase fruit, vegetable, and low-fat dairy products • Antihypertensive therapy on an individual basis
Abnormal lipid profile	Total cholesterol level < 4.5 mmol/L (175 mg/dl) Low density lipids < 2.5 mmol/L (100 mg/dl)	• Dietary modification: reduced fat intake (supplemental omega-3 fatty acids) • Lifestyle modification: weight control and exercise • Lipid lowering agents: statin $+/-$ fibrate
Sedentary lifestyle	Minimum of 30 minutes moderate to high intensity exercise 3–4 times per week	• Assess risk of potential adverse effects (much lower than often predicted) • Self-motivated programs around daily activities • Formal exercise programs
Overweight/obesity*	Body mass index 18.5 to 24.9 kg/m^2 Waist circumference: < 100 cm in men and < 90 cm in women	• Self-motivated program • Dietary modification (as above) • Lifestyle modification (as above) • Formal exercise programs • Formal dietary management programs
Diabetes/metabolic syndrome*	$HbA1_c < 7\%$	• Dietary management • Optimize exercise and lipid profile • Hypoglycemic therapy
Preventative pharmacologic therapies	Antiplatelet therapy	• Aspirin 75 to 325 mg/day in majority of patients • Clopidogrel 75mg/day • Warfarin titrated to INR of 2.0 to 3.0
	ACE inhibitors	• Chronic therapy titrated to highest therapeutic dose in all patients with coronary heart disease: unequivocal recommendation in those with diabetes or left ventricular systolic dysfunction
	Beta-blockers	• Chronic therapy in those with an ACS

of cardiorespiratory disease. The following sections summarize and interpret (as will be noted in Chapter 7, it is important to consult the latest detailed guidelines in developing protocols) therapeutic targets specific to each of these conditions: remembering that any attempts to accommodate the "cookbook" approach offered by expert guidelines becomes progressively harder to apply with competing therapeutic priorities and the needs of the individual [176]. Ultimately, the clinical support and management of affected patients has to take into account those symptoms that most affect them in conjunction with any consequences (i.e. reduced survival) derived from selecting specific therapeutic targets.

> The following therapeutic targets in relation to optimizing outcomes in chronic angina pectoris are largely based on the following guidelines:
>
> Task Force of the European Society of Cardiology. Management of stable angina pectoris. *Eur Heart J* 1997; **18**:394–413.
>
> Mannheimer C, Camici P, Chester MR, et al., on behalf of The Joint Study Group on the treatment of refractory angina. The problem of chronic refractory angina. *Eur Heart J* 2002; **23**:355–370.
>
> Gibbon RJ, Abrams J, Chatterjee K, et al., on behalf of The ACC/AHA Task Force on Practice Guidelines (Committee on the management of patients with chronic stable angina). ACC/AHA 2002 Guideline update for the management of patients with chronic stable angina – summary article. *Circulation* 2003; **107**:149–158.

Key therapeutic targets in chronic angina pectoris

A large proportion of the recommendations relating to those affected by chronic angina pectoris are consistent with the therapeutic targets relating to secondary prevention outlined in Table 2.1. Other than addressing the traditional risk factors at the individual level (e.g. smoking and hypertension), it is clear that the emerging role of the "metabolic syndrome" (comprising a number interrelated risk factors and pathological processes) has assumed increasing importance in slowing the progression of coronary artery disease: the concept of "absolute" versus "relative" risk, whereby the combined presence of risk factors is used to calculate the probability (in absolute percentage terms) of a coronary event (fatal or otherwise) occurring with a defined period (usually 10 years). In terms of the active management of this condition, there are three key therapeutic targets or goals:

1 *Accurately determine the extent of the disease.* Coronary angiography remains the gold standard method for determining the presence and extent of the disease. However, a number of investigations including 12-lead ECG, ECG stress testing, ambulatory EGC monitoring, echocardiography (both at rest and stress echocardiography) and nuclear imaging techniques, provide further information concerning the extent of myocardial ischemia, its effects

on myocardial function and, importantly, whether or not revascularization (in the form of coronary angioplasty or coronary artery bypass) will address areas of reversible ischemia (i.e. stunned or hibernating myocardium) as opposed to those areas with fixed perfusion defects or myocardial necrosis.

2 *Optimal pharmacotherapy.* Consistent with the recommendations outlined in Table 2.1 all patients with chronic angina pectoris should have their lipid profile and subsequent suitability for dietary modification and/or prescribed statin therapy assessed in addition to the application of antiplatelet therapy. The three major classes of drug used to reduce the extent of myocardial ischemia and, therefore, anginal symptoms are nitrates (both in terms of acute sublingual therapy for angina pectoris on exertion and as chronic therapy in the form of longer-acting preparations), beta-blockers and calcium antagonists. As noted by the ACC/AHA expert committee, all three forms of pharmacotherapy in appropriate doses can be effectively used to limit anginal symptoms. However, individual variability in respect to both their beneficial and potential adverse effects is common.

3 *Revascularization.* Given an accurate determination of the extent of ischemia and its reversible component, there is a clear role for revascularization – particularly when there are target lesions that can be targeted via a coronary artery bypass or, more frequently in recent years, via percutaneous transluminal coronary angioplasty with the additional use of a drug-eluting stent designed to reduce reocclusion by inhibiting local thrombus formation and fibrosis.

Despite meeting many of the therapeutic goals and targets outlined above, a significant proportion of individuals suffer from chronic refractory angina. Moreover, given the fact that current therapeutics (despite their short-term efficacy) do not address the underlying progression of the disease with age (and contributory conditions) and the progressive ageing of the population, will no doubt lead to an increased number of affected individuals. It is within this context that in the past few years there has been consideration of a new and "novel" range of pharmacologic agents to combat this condition. In particular novel "metabolic" agents that appear to have an "oxygen-sparing" effect and therefore minimize underlying myocardial ischemia appear to markedly improve anginal symptoms in those with refractory angina pectoris. For example, perhexiline an antianginal agent that was first introduced in the 1970s but discarded in the 1980s has been recently reintroduced in patients with refractory angina due to a better understanding of its complex pharmacodynamic and pharmacokinetic profile and safer use of the drug via therapeutic drug monitoring [177]. Perhexiline acts prophylactically in chronic refractory angina via the inhibition of a key enzyme involved in normal cardiac metabolism [178]. This inhibition leads to a change in myocardial metabolism substrate selection from free-fatty acids to glucose. This change improves cardiac efficiency, by reducing oxygen demand and removing intracellular toxins [178]. This "new old" drug has proved to be the forerunner of a range of other "metabolic" agents including trimetazidine, ranolazine, and etomoxir [179].

Note: The metabolic syndrome is defined by the ACC/AHA as the combination of abdominal obesity, abnormal lipid profile (i.e. elevated total cholesterol level and abnormal high versus low density lipid level), hypertension and elevated serum glucose levels.

> The following therapeutic targets in relation to optimizing outcomes in CHF are largely based on the following guidelines:
>
> Swedberg K, Cleland J, Dargie H, Drexler H, Follath F, on behalf of the Task Force for the Diagnosis and Treatment of Chronic Heart Failure of the European Society of Cardiology Guidelines for the diagnosis and treatment of chronic heart failure: executive summary (update 2005): The Task Force for the Diagnosis and Treatment of Chronic Heart Failure of the European Society of Cardiology. *Eur Heart J* 2005; **26**(11):1115–1140.
>
> Hunt SA, Baker DW, Chin MH, Cinquegrani MP, Feldman AM, on behalf of the American College of Cardiology/American Heart Association Task Force on Practice Guidelines (Committee to Revise the 1995 Guidelines for the evaluation and management of heart failure); International Society for Heart and Lung Transplantation; Heart Failure Society of America ACC/AHA Guidelines for the evaluation and management of chronic heart failure in the adult: executive summary a report of the American College of Cardiology/American Heart Association Task Force on Practice Guidelines (Committee to Revise the 1995 Guidelines for the evaluation and management of heart failure). Developed in collaboration with the International Society for Heart and Lung Transplantation; endorsed by the Heart Failure Society of America. *Circulation* 2001; **104**(24):2996–3007.
>
> Krum, H., Jelinek, M., Stewart, S., Sindone, A., Hawkes, A., Atherton, J. On behalf of the National Heart Foundation of Australia and Cardiac Society of Australia and New Zealand Chronic Heart Failure Clinical Practice Guidelines Expert Writing Panel. Guidelines for the Prevention, Detection and Management of People with Chronic Heart Failure in Australia, 2006.

Key therapeutic targets in chronic heart failure

There is little doubt that the complexity of CHF and concurrent disease states that usually complicate its management (see the next section on AF as an example!) means that optimizing the management of this syndrome is extremely challenging. As the frequent "bridge" between the first signs of chronic cardiac disease and death, the purpose and direction of that management can rapidly change. Consistent with this book's consistent emphasis on secondary prevention and delaying the progression of the underlying pathology, it is relevant to refer to the recent update of the AHA/ACC guidelines for the management of CHF. In response to the evolving epidemiologic profile of this syndrome, this expert committee proposed a more proactive way to classify and tackle a sustained epidemic of CHF. As such, they identified four key stages of heart failure with the following features:

Stage A   Individuals at high-risk of developing heart failure: those with pre-existing hypertension, coronary artery disease, left bundle branch block, diabetes and a body mass index of > 30 kg/m^2 (obesity).

Stage B   Individuals with previous AMI, asymptomatic valvular disease, and/or asymptomatic left ventricular systolic dysfunction (so-called asymptomatic or "latent" heart failure).

Stage C   Individuals with symptomatic heart failure (CHF).

Stage D   Patients with severe CHF who have been admitted to hospital.

Once an individual has developed CHF (i.e. a symptomatic form of heart failure), there are a range of therapeutic targets that, if achieved, will *potentially* improve quality of life, reduce morbidity and prolong the life of the affected individual (remembering that there is no cure for CHF). These include:

1 *Accurately determine the presence and extent of the syndrome.* Although there is an evolving role for screening "at risk" individuals via elevated brain natriuretic peptide levels, diagnosis of CHF is based on the combination of clinical features, chest radiography in the acute phase, and objective measurement of ventricular function (most commonly echocardiography) to determine the presence of left ventricular systolic dysfunction or abnormal filling pressures or relaxation indicative of "diastolic heart failure" in the absence of systolic dysfunction. Consistent with the management of chronic angina pectoris, there is also a clear role for nuclear cardiological testing, stress echocardiography, and positron emission tomography to assess potential reversibility of ischemia and viability of myocardium in those with concurrent evidence of active coronary heart disease.

2 *Optimal pharmacotherapy.* Angiotensin-converting enzyme (ACE) inhibitors (e.g. enalapril) are the cornerstones of pharmacological therapy to prevent disease progression and prolong survival. Similarly, beta-blockers (e.g. carvedilol) prolong survival when added to ACE inhibitors in symptomatic patients. Diuretics (predominantly loop diuretics) provide symptom relief and restoration or maintenance of euvolemia in those individuals who experience cardiopulmonary congestion (as demonstrated by pulmonary or peripheral edema). In those with more advanced CHF (i.e. remain symptomatic despite the application of ACE inhibitors and beta-blockers), digoxin and spironolactone, angiotensin II receptor antagonists (e.g. candersartan), and digoxin have the potential to improve quality of life, prevent morbidity, and prolong survival.

3 *Adjunctive device therapy.* Biventricular pacing may have a role in those individuals in NYHA functional Class III or IV with wide QRS complexes in improving exercise tolerance and quality of life. Moreover, implantable cardioverter defibrillators have been shown to reduce the risk of sudden cardiac death (a major cause of death) in patients with CHF and severe systolic dysfunction of the left ventricle. Pacing may be needed to treat symptomatic bradyarrhythmias and/or sick-sinus syndrome. If possible, atrioventricular

synchrony should be maintained due to the significant contribution of atrial filling to cardiac output in CHF. Upgrading a ventricular pacemaker to a dual-chamber device should be considered in patients with CHF who have maintained sinus rhythm.

4 *Optimal nonpharmacological strategies.* A range of adjunctive strategies can be used to improve the quality of life of affected individuals and, potentially, avoid clinical crises and prolong survival. These include careful fluid management: wherever possible, determine the patient's ideal "dry or euvolemic" weight (when a patient who has had signs of fluid retention after diuretic treatment reaches a steady weight at which there are no further signs of fluid overload). Using this ideal weight as a goal, encourage patients to weigh themselves daily, record it in a diary and adjust their fluid intake and use of diuretic therapy (as a flexible regimen) accordingly. As malnutrition, cardiac cachexia, and anemia are common problems that contribute to the debilitating symptoms of weakness and fatigue associated with CHF-affected individuals need to be thoroughly investigated for the underlying cause (e.g. intestinal malabsorption due to chronic ischemia, hepatomegaly, or iron-deficiency) and referred to specialist dietary intervention/nutritional support via a qualified dietician (e.g. to be prescribed a specific sodium restricted diet plus supplemental vitamins). Contrary to conventional thinking, there are also theoretical benefits of promoting exercise in CHF to reverse associated deconditioning of peripheral and respiratory muscles in addition to improving endothelial function. Meta-analyses demonstrate that inhospital and home exercise training programs for CHF can be successfully applied without significant adverse effects. Improved outcomes associated with reported programs include increased exercise capacity, decreased resting catecholamines, improved heart rate variability and, most importantly, quality of life.

The following therapeutic targets in relation to optimizing outcomes in AF are largely based on the following guidelines:

American College of Cardiology/American Heart Association Task Force on Practice Guidelines and the European Society of Cardiology Committee for Practice Guidelines and Policy Conferences (Committee to Develop Guidelines for the management of patients with atrial fibrillation). ACC/AHA/ESC Guidelines for the management of patients with atrial fibrillation: executive summary. *Circulation* 2001; **104**:2118–2150.

Key therapeutic targets in atrial fibrillation

Because AF typically emerges in much older individuals in whom chronic cardiac disease is already well established, there is a natural temptation to concentrate solely on passively controlling this arrhythmia. However, as emphasized in the previous sections, unless there has been a conscious decision to adopt a palliative approach, there are strong clinical and pathological reasons why *proactively* targeting the typical precursors and risk factors that "drive" AF: particularly in terms of preventing "malignant" paroxysmal events and/or increasing the likelihood of the underlying cardiac rhythm evolving into persistent AF.

It is within this context that there are three overriding principles that underpin the management of AF:

1 Reestablish normal sinus rhythm.

2 If unable to permanently reestablish normal sinus rhythm, minimize the absolute time spent in AF and aggressively control the underlying ventricular rate.*

3 Minimize the thromboembolic risk imposed by AF.

Unfortunately, all three are difficult to achieve given the combination of the typical age of affected individuals, the need for close surveillance/monitoring, the fine line associated with the risk-benefits provided by current therapeutics and the presence of confounding comorbidities. In terms of the active management of this arrhythmia, there are a number of therapeutic targets or goals:

1 *Accurately determine what form of AF is present.* An immediate diagnosis of AF requires documentation of a single-lead ECG. However, vital information (e.g. LV hypertrophy, bundle branch block) is gained from a 12-lead ECG. If there is evidence of sporadic events or indeed a more permanent form of AF, a 24-hour Holter monitor should be applied and carefully analyzed. Additional electrophysiology studies, where appropriate, will determine whether of not the arrhythmia can be terminated (e.g. via an ablation procedure), clarify the mechanism of an associated wide QRS-complex tachycardia and identify any predisposing arrhythmias such as paroxysmal supraventricular tachycardia. Similarly, exercise testing can provide vital information in terms of an "inducible" component with exercise and/or the adequacy of ventricular rate control.

2 *Determine the extent of thromboembolic risk.* Given the close association between AF and stroke, it important to categorize the risk of a future thromboembolic event. Overall, individuals with nonvalvular AF have a six-fold increased risk of thromboembolism: the major risk factors for an ischemic stroke and systemic embolism being prior history of the same, hypertension, CHF, advancing age (particularly beyond 65 years of age), diabetes and coronary artery disease. In this context, transesophageal echocardiography is also vital to determine the presence of thrombus in the left atrial appendage

---

*There is still debate concerning the relative merits of aggressively controlling the ventricular rate in AF versus administering potentially toxic pharmacologic agents to maintain sinus rhythm. This issue further emphasizes the need for individually tailored management.

(this is a contraindication for electrical cardioversion). As thyrotoxicosis also increases the risk of AF and resistance to cardioversion, thyroid function should also be routinely assessed and appropriately managed. Any individual aged 65 years or more with any of the above risk factors should be considered as "high risk" in this regard.

3 *Determine the extent of associated cardiac dysfunction.* A range of other standard cardiorespiratory investigations, including chest radiography and transthoracic echocardiography should be used to determine any contributory cardiac abnormalities (e.g. valvular dysfunction, left ventricular systolic dysfunction, and chronic respiratory disease).

4 *Converting the AF to sinus rhythm.* This can be attempted with either electrical or pharmacological cardioversion: the latter appears to be more efficacious when initiated within seven days of the onset of AF and the former is particularly indicated in paroxysmal AF associated with a rapid ventricular response and a hemodynamic/ischemic crisis. Within seven days of onset, the most effective agents include dofetilide (a Type III antiarrhythmic that is also effective when applied to more prolonged AF), flecanide, ibutilide, and propafenone.

5 *Maintaining sinus rhythm.* There is a range of pharmacological agents used to maintain sinus rhythm, once achieved. These include sotalol, amiodarone, and dofetilide. The major consideration is risk-benefit based on the number of concurrent disease states/precipitants that may trigger new episodes of AF, the extent of cardiac compromise associated with these events and the safety profile and, indeed, individual response to the selected agent.

6 *Controlling the ventricular rate in persistent or permanent AF.* If the ventricular rate is elevated beyond normal physiologic parameters (after a careful assessment of the underlying ventricular rate both at rest and during exercise), a beta-blocker or calcium antagonist should be prescribed. Digoxin is indicated in those patients with concurrent left ventricular systolic dysfunction.

7 *Reducing the risk of subsequent thromboembolic events.* All patients (excepting younger individuals with "lone" AF) should receive either antiplatelet (i.e. aspirin) or anticoagulation (i.e. warfarin) therapy. Given the narrow therapeutic margins associated with warfarin (with the need for regular monitoring of INRs to maintain levels of 2.0 to 3.0 in those aged < 75 years and 1.6 to 2.5 in older individuals) with increased risk of bleeding events (e.g. intracranial hemorrhage), a careful assessment based on risk (see above) should be used to decide whether aspirin is a more appropriate agent in this regard.

2.4 Dying from cardiac disease: optimizing the of end-of-life

Not surprisingly, the advanced stages of chronic cardiac disease can have a devastating effect on a patient's quality of life. Unfortunately, many patients with nonmalignant disease states have little or no access to palliative care programs. Nor are potentially useful palliative strategies applied. These issues have been particularly highlighted in relation to CHF, but apply equally to those dying from other forms of heart disease. The reasons for the absence of palliative care services include a lack of resources and expertise, and problems associated with determining prognosis.

Guiding principles of management

Predicting the illness trajectory in patients with end-stage CHF and other forms chronic cardiac disease is much harder when compared to those with terminal malignancy. This creates uncertainty and can potentially prevent doctors telling patients when they have reached the terminal phase of their illness and from planning appropriate care. The emerging literature surrounding this subject, particularly in relation to CHF, clearly identifies the following goals of management in this context:

1 Availability of protocols for the management of end-stage/refractory heart disease to ensure that a reversible component of the disease process has not been overlooked, and that all reasonable treatment options have been considered.

2 Clear guidelines to determine when it is appropriate to talk to the patient and their family/carers about the prospect of death and their preferences in this regard (e.g. advanced directives and living wills). It has been suggested that any individual considered to be at high risk of dying within 12 months should be considered for palliation.

3 Identifying the most appropriate management to provide quality end-of-life (i.e. symptom relief, diuretics, pain control).

4 Identifying what is inappropriate management (i.e. inotropes, dialysis, central lines, artificial ventilation and urinary catheters – unless the patient has a retention or for his/her comfort not just to monitor urinary output).

5 Good coordination and continuity of care by a single health care professional.

Key therapeutic targets in terminal chronic cardiac disease

There are very few guidelines to facilitate the optimal management of those dying from terminal cardiac disease. However, it is reasonable to suggest the following therapeutic targets in this context:

1 Effective communication between the health care team, the patient and their family/carers (where appropriate) to determine the patient's health care and quality of life priorities at the end-of-life.

2 Supportive management to maintain the patient's independence as long as possible.

3 Adequate analgesia and other palliative care strategies to minimize pain and discomfort.

4 Psychological support and counseling to minimize emotional and psychological distress.

5 A peaceful death!

2.5 Summary

The combined pages of expert recommendations and opinion used to derive the key therapeutic targets listed above number more than *one hundred* and the studies and papers on which they are based in the *thousands*. Unfortunately, this does not mean that we know exactly what to do in order to fully attenuate the impact of chronic cardiac disease on quality of life, morbidity and premature mortality. However, there is a growing recognition that if we were to spend as much time applying what we know now, as opposed to generating new therapeutic options (i.e. freezing "curative" research in favor of "translational" research), we would be able to make a substantial impact on the individual and societal burden imposed by common disease states such as chronic cardiac disease. Certainly, there is ample evidence to suggest that "malignant" conditions such as CHF [180] and AF [181] are routinely undertreated and mismanaged. This first section of the book has attempted, therefore, to firstly establish the size of the problem in relation to chronic cardiac disease and, secondly, outline what can be done to subsequently improve health outcomes. The remaining sections of the book will subsequent examine the individual and organizational factors that further influence health outcomes in relation to chronic cardiac disease (Section 2), the evidence in favor of programs of care that have the potential to both delay the progression and severity of the disease and successfully improve day-to-day management of symptomatic patients (Section 3), before bringing together all the aspects of the preceding sections to describe what is most likely to be cost-effective when establishing a service targeting individuals affected by chronic cardiac disease (Section 4).

References

1 Yusuf S, Reddy S, Onupuu S, et al. Global burden of cardiovascular diseases: part I: general considerations, the epidemiologic transition, risk factors and impact of urbanisation. *Circulation* 2001; **104**:2746–2753.

2 Yusuf S, Reddy S, Ounupuu S, et al. Global burden of cardiovascular diseases, part II: variations in cardiovascular disease by specific ethnic groups and geographic regions and prevention strategies. *Circulation* 2001; **104**:2855–2864.

3 Murray CJL, Lopez AD, eds. *The global burden of disease: a comprehensive assessment of mortality and disability from disease, injuries, and risk factors in 1990 and projected to 2020.* Boston, MA: Harvard School of Public Health, 1996.

4 Omran AR. The epidemiological transition: a theory of the epidemiology of population change. *Milbank Mem Fund Q* 1971; **49**:509–538.

5 World Health Organisation. *Atlas of heart disease & stroke* (Chapter 13, Global burden of coronary heart disease). Geneva: World Health Organisation, 2005. http://www.who.int/cardiovascular_diseases/resources/atlas/en/print.html. Accessed June 2005.

6 Lloyd-Jones DM, Larson MG, Alexa B, et al. Lifetime risk of developing coronary heart disease. *Lancet* 1999; **353**:89–92.

7 Henry K, Melroe H, Huebsch J, et al. Severe premature coronary artery disease with protease inhibitors. *Lancet* 1998; **351**:1328.

8 Hsue PY, Giri K, Erickson S, et al. Clinical features of acute coronary syndromes in patients with human immunodeficiency virus infection. *Circulation* 2004; **109**:316–319.

9 United Nations world population prospects: the 1998 revision. 2005. Accessed online 21 June 2005. http://www.abs.gov.au/Ausstats/abs@.nsf/Lookup/93D90E2E55DFA003CA256A7100188A7C

10 Carroll K, Majeed A, Firth C, et al. Prevalence and management of coronary heart disease in primary care: population-based cross-sectional study using a disease register. *J Public Health* 2003; **25**:29–35.

11 Knopp RH. Risk factors for CAD in women. *Am J Cardiol* 2002; **89**:28E–35E.

12 Kannel WB, Feinleib M, McNamara PM, et al. An investigation of heart disease in families: the Framingham Offspring Study. *Am J Epidemiol* 1979; **110**:281–290.

13 Bhopal R, Hayes L, White M, et al. Ethnic and socio-economic inequalities in coronary heart disease, diabetes and risk factors in Europeans and South Asians. *J Public Health Med* 2002; **24**(2):95–105.

14 Rutter MK, Meigs JB, Sullivan LM, et al. C-reactive protein, the metabolic syndrome, and prediction of cardiovascular events in the Framingham Offspring Study. *Circulation* 2004; **110**:380–385.

15 Pearson TA, Mensah GA, Alexander RW, et al. Markers of inflammation and cardiovascular disease. *Circulation* 2003; **107**:499–511.

16 Hoffman JI, Kaplan S, Liberthson RR. Prevalence of congenital heart disease. *Am Heart J* 2004;**147**(3):398–400.

17 Bostom AG, Silbershatz H, Rosenberg IH, et al. Nonfasting plasma total homocysteine levels and all-cause and cardiovascular disease mortality in elderly Framingham men and women. *Arch Intern Med* 1999; **159**:1077–1080.

18 Bunker SJ, Colquhoun DM, Esler MD, et al. "Stress" and coronary heart disease: psychosocial risk factors. National Heart Foundation of Australia position statement update. *Med J Aust* 2003; **178**:272–276.

19 Wells AJ. Passive smoking as a cause of heart disease. *J Am Coll Cardiol* 1994; **24**:546–554.

20 Kannel WB, Feinleb M. Natural history coronary of angina pectoris in the Framingham Study. Prognosis and survival. *Am J Cardiol* 1972; **29**:154–163.

21 Voss R, Cullen P, Schulte H, et al. Prediction of risk of coronary events in middle-aged men in the Prospective Cardiovascular Munster Study (PROCAM) using neural networks. *Int J Epidemiol* 2002; **31**:1253–1262.

22 Salomaa V, Keonen M, Koukkunen H, et al. Decline in out-of-hospital coronary heart disease deaths has contributed the main part to the overall decline in coronary heart disease mortality rates among persons 35 to 64 years of age in Finland. *Circulation* 2003; **10**:691–696.

23 Long-term Intervention with Pravastatin in Ischaemic Disease (LIPID) Study Group. Prevention of cardiovascular events and death with pravastatin in patients with coronary heart disease and a broad range of initial cholesterol levels. *N Engl J Med* 1998; **339**:1349–1357.

24 Downs JR, Clearfield M, Weis S, et al. Primary prevention of acute coronary events with lovastatin in men and women with average cholesterol levels. Results of AFCAPS/TexCAPS. *JAMA* 1998; **279**:1615–1622.

25 Ballantyne C, Arroll B, Shepherd J. Lipids and CVD management: towards a global consensus. *Eur Heart J* 2005 (E-pub Jun 21): In press.
26 Karpe F, Boquist S, Tang R, et al. Remnant lipoproteins are related to intima-media thickness of the carotid artery independently of LDL cholesterol and plasma triglycerides. *J Lipid Res* 2001; **42**:17–21.
27 Hamsten A, Silveira A, Boquist S, et al. The Apolipoprotein CI content of triglyceride-rich lipoproteins independently predicts early atherosclerosis in healthy middle-aged men. *J Am Coll Cardiol* 2005; **45**:1013–1017.
28 Walldius G, Junger I, Holme I, et al. High apolipoprotein B, low apolipoprotien A-I, and improvement in the prediction of fatal myocardial infarction (AMORIS) study: a prospective study. *Lancet* 2001; **358**:2026–2033.
29 American Heart Association – National and international statistics. Accessed online 15 June 2005. http://www.americanheart.org/downloadable/heart/1105390918119HDSStats2005Update.pdf
30 Chobanian AV, Bakris GL, Black HR, et al. and the National high blood pressure education program coordinating committee. The seventh report of the joint national committee on prevention, detection, evaluation and treatment of high blood pressure: The JNC 7 Report. *JAMA* 2003; **289**:2560–2572.
31 The American Heart Association 2005: Diabetes http://www.americanheart.org/presenter.jhtml?identifier=4546. Accessed June 2005.
32 British Heart Foundation Coronary Heart Disease Statistics. Accessed online June 25 2005. http://www.bhf.org.uk/professionals/index.asp?secondlevel=519
33 Liese AD, Schulz M, Moore CG, et al. Dietary patterns, insulin sensitivity and adiposity in the multi-ethnic insulin resistance atherosclerosis study population. *Br J Nutr* 2004; **92**:973–84.
34 Vasan RS, Sullivan LM, Wilson PF, et al. Relative importance of borderline and elevated levels of coronary heart disease risk factors. *Ann Intern Med* 2005; **142**:393–402.
35 Marsh SA, Coombs JS. Exercise and the endothelial cell. *Int J Cardiol* 2005; **99**(2):165–169.
36 Spencer CG, Martin SC, Felmeden DC, et al. Relationship of homocysteine to markers of platelet and endothelial activation in "high risk" hypertensives: a substudy of the Anglo-Scandinavian Cardiac Outcomes Trial. *Int J Cardiol.* 2004; **94**:293–300.
37 Agatisa PK, Mathews KA, Bromberger JT, et al. Coronary and aortic calcification in women with a history of major depression. *Arch Intern Med* 2005; **165**(11):1229–1236.
38 Onupuu S, Negassa A, Yusuf S., for the INTERHEART Investigators. Effect of potentially modifiable risk factors associated with myocardial infarction in 52 countries (the INTERHEART study): case-control study. *Lancet* 2004; **364**:937–952.
39 Rosengren A, Hawken S, Ounpuu S, et al. for the INTERHEART Investigators. Association of psychosocial risk factors with risk of acute myocardial infarction in 11 119 cases and 13,648 controls from 52 countries (the INTERHEART Study): case control study. *Lancet* 2004; **364**:953–962.
40 MacIntyre K, Stewart S, Capewell S, et al. Heart of inequality – the relationship between socio-economic deprivation and death from a first acute myocardial infarction: a population-based analysis. *BMJ* 2001; **322**: 1152–1153.
41 Wilson DK, Kirtland KA, Ainsworth BE, et al. Socioeconomic status and perceptions of access and safety for physical activity. *Ann Behav Med* 2004; **28**(1):20–28.

42 Bos V, Kunst AE, Garssen J, et al. Socioecconomic inequalities within ethnic groups in The Netherlands, 1995–2000. *J Epidemiol Community Health* 2005; **59**(4):329–335.

43 Pekkanen J, Uutela A, Valkonen T, et al. Coronary risk factor levels: differences between educational groups in 1972–87 in eastern Finland. *J. Epidemiol Community Health* 1995; **49**:144–149.

44 Tenconi MT, Devoti G, Comelli M, and RIFLE research group. Role of socioeconomic indicators in the prediction of all causes and coronary heart disease mortality in over 12,000 men – the Italian RIFLE pooling project. *Eur J Epidemiol* 2000; **16**:565–571.

45 Kim MC, Kini A, Sharma SK. Refractory angina pectoris mechanism and therapeutic options. *J Am Coll Cardiol* 2002; **39**(6):923–934.

46 Gibbons RJ, Abrams J, Chatterjee K, et al. ACC/AHA 2002 Guideline update for the management of patients with chronic stable angina – summary article. A report of the American College of Cardiology/American Heart Association Task Force on Practice Guidelines (Committee on the management of patients with chronic stable angina). *Circulation* 2003; **107**:149–158.

47 European Society of Cardiology Guidelines on the management of stable angina pectoris. Recommendation of the task force of the European Society of Cardiology. *Eur Heart J* 1997; **18**:394–413.

48 Abrams J. Chronic stable angina. *New Engl J Med* 2005; **352**:2524–2533.

49 Mannheimer C, Camici P, Chester MR, et al. The problem of chronic refractory angina. Report from the ESC Joint Study Group on the treatment of refractory angina. *Eur Heart J* 2002; **23**:355–370.

50 Stewart S. Refractory to medical treatment but not to nursing care: can we do more for patients with chronic angina pectoris? *Eur J Cardiov Nursing* 2003; **2**:169–170.

51 Lewin RJ. Improving quality of life in patients with angina. *Heart* 1999; **82**:654–655.

52 Lewin RJ, Furze G, Robinson J, et al. A randomised controlled trial of a self-management plan for patients with newly diagnosed angina. *Br J Gen Pract* 2002; **52**:194–201.

53 Campeau L. Grading of angina pectoris (letter). *Circulation* 1976; **54**:522–523.

54 Bertrand ME, Simoons ML, Fox KAA, et al. Management of acute coronary syndromes: acute coronary syndromes without persistent ST segment elevation. Recommendations of the Task Force of the European Society of Cardiology. *Eur Heart J* 2000; **21**:1406–1432.

55 Rose GA. The diagnosis of ischaemic heart pain and intermittent claudication in field surveys. *Bull World Health Organ* 1962; **27**:645–658.

56 Jackson G. Clinical benefits of a metabolic approach to the management of coronary patients. *Eur Heart J Suppl* 1999 **1**:O28–O31.

57 Stary HC, Chandler AB, Glagov S, et al. A definition of initial, fatty streak, and intermediate lesions of atherosclerosis. A report from the committee on vascular lesions of the Council on Arteriosclerosis, American Heart Association. *Circulation* 1994; **89**:2462–2478.

58 Ross R. The Pathogenesis of atherosclerosis: a perspective for the 1990s. *Nature* 1993; **362**:801–809.

59 McGill HC, McMahan CA, Herderick EE, et al. Origin of atherosclerosis in childhood and adolescence. *Am J Clin Nutr* 2000; **72**(5):1307S–1315S.

60 Kavey RM, Daniels SR, Lauer RM, et al. American Heart Association Guidelines for Primary prevention of atherosclerotic cardiovascular disease beginning in childhood. *Circulation* 2003; **107**:1562–1566.

61 Stary HC, Chandler AB, Glagov S, et al. A definition of advanced types of atherosclerotic lesions and a histological classification of atherosclerosis. A report from the Committee on vascular lesions of the council on arteriosclerosis, American Heart Association. *Arterioscler Thromb Vasc Biol* 1995; **15**:1512–1531.

62 Davies MJ, Thomas A. Thrombosis and acute coronary-artery lesions in sudden cardiac ischaemic death. *N Engl J Med* 1984;**310**(18):1137–1140.

63 Stanley WC, Recchia FA, Lopaschuk GD. Myocardial substrate metabolism in the normal and failing heart. *Physiol Rev* 2005; **85**:1093–1129.

64 Stanley WC, Chandler MP. Energy metabolism in the normal and failing heart: potential for therapeutic interventions. *Heart Fail Rev* 2002; **7**(24):115–130.

65 Lee L, Horowitz JD, Frenneaux M. Metabolic manipulation in ischaemic heart disease, a novel approach to treatment. *Eur Heart J* 2004; **25**(7):634–641.

66 Lopaschuk GD, Belke DD, Gamble J, et al. Regulation of fatty acid oxidation in the mammalian heart in health and disease. *Biochim Biophys Acta* 1994; **1213**:263–276.

67 Liedtke, AJ. Alterations of carbohydrate and lipid metabolism in the acutely ischaemic heart. *Prog Cardiovasc Dis* 1981; **23**(5):321–336.

68 Stanley WC. Partial fatty acid oxidation inhibitors for stable angina. *Expert Opin Investig Drugs* 2002; **11**(5):615–629.

69 Taegtmeyer H, Roberts AF, Raine AE. Energy metabolism in reperfused heart muscle: metabolic correlates to return of function. *J Am Coll Cardiol* 1985; **6**(4):864–870.

70 Depre C, Vanoverschelde JL, Taegtmeyer H. Glucose for the heart. *Circulation* 1999; **99**(4):578–588.

71 Lampe FC, Whincup PH, Wannamethee SG, et al. The natural history of prevalent ischaemic heart disease in middle-aged men. *Eur Heart J* 2000; **21**:1052–1062.

72 Hemingway H, Shipley M, Britton A, et al. Prognosis of angina with and without a diagnosis: 11-year follow-up in the Whitehall II prospective cohort study. *BMJ* 2003; **327**:895.

73 Rose G, Hamilton PS, Keen H, et al. Myocardial ischaemia, risk factors and death from coronary heart disease. *Lancet* 1977; **1**:105–109.

74 Murphy NF, Stewart S, Hart CL, et al. A population study of the long-term consequences of angina: 20 year follow-up of the Renfrew-Paisley study. *Submitted for publication.*

75 Sigurdsson E, Sigfusson N, Agnarsson U, et al. Long-term prognosis of different forms of coronary heart disease: the Reykjavik Study. *Int J Epidemiol* 1995; **24**:58–68.

76 Rosengren A, Wilhelmsen L, Hagman M, et al. Natural history of myocardial infarction and angina pectoris in a general population sample of middle-aged men: a 16-year follow-up of the Primary Prevention Study, Goteborg, Sweden. *J Intern Med* 1998; **244**:495–505.

77 Wood P. *Diseases of the Heart and Circulation*. London: Chapman and Hall, 1968.

78 Braunwald E, Grossman W. Clinical aspects of heart failure. In: Braunwald E, ed. *Heart Disease*, 4th edn. New York: WB Saunders,1992, p. 444.

79 Packer M. Survival in patients with chronic heart failure and its potential modification by drug therapy. In: Cohn J, ed. *Drug Treatment of Heart Failure*, 2nd edn. Secaucus, New Jersey: ATC International, 1988, p. 273.

80 Poole-Wilson PA. Changing ideas in the treatment of heart failure: an overview *Cardiology* 1987; **74**:53–7

81 Hunt SA, Baker Dw, Chin MH, et al. ACC/AHA guidelines for the evaluation and management of chronic heart failure in the adult. A report of the American College of Cardiology/American Heart Association Task Force on practice guidelines. (Committee to revise the 1995 guidelines for the evaluation and management of heart failure) 2001. Accessed online 29 June 2005. http://www.acc.org/clinical/guidelines/failure/II_characterization.htm#II_A

82 Swedburg K, Cleland J, Dargie H, et al. ESC Guidelines for the diagnosis and treatment of chronic heart failure: executive summary (update 2005). The Task Force for the diagnosis and treatment of CHF of the European Society of Cardiology. *Eur Heart J* 2005; **26**:1115–1140.

83 Krum H, Gilbert RE. Demographics and concomitant disorders in heart failure. *Lancet* 2003; **362**:147–158.

84 Krum H, Jelinek M, Stewart S, Sindone A, Hawkes A, Atherton J. On behalf of the National Heart Foundation of Australia and Cardiac Society of Australia and New Zealand Chronic Heart Failure Clinical Practice Guidelines Expert Writing Panel. Guidelines for the Prevention, Detection and Management of People with Chronic Heart Failure in Australia, 2006.

85 Brixius K, Reuter H, Bloch W, et al. Altered hetero- and homeometric autoregulation in the terminally failing human heart. *Eur J Heart Fail* 2005; **7**:29–35.

86 Taylor MR, Bristow MR. The emerging pharmacogenomics of the beta-adrenergic receptors. *Congest Heart Fail* 2004; **10**:281–288.

87 Narula J, Kolodgie FD, Virmani R. Apoptosis and cardiomyopathy. *Curr Opin Cardiol* 2000; **15**(3): 183–188.

88 Schrier RW, Abraham WT. Mechanisms of disease: hormones and hemodynamics in heart failure. *N Engl J Med* 1999; **341**(8): 577–585.

89 Suresh DP, Lamba S, Abraham WT. New developments in heart failure: role of endothelin and the use of endothelin receptor antagonists. *J Card Fail* 2000; **6**(4): 359–368.

90 Blum A, Miller H. Pathophysiological role of cytokines in congestive heart failure. *Ann Rev Med* 2001; **52**:15–27.

91 Aukrust P, Gullestad L, Ueland, Damas JK, Yndestad A. Inflammatory and anti-inflammatory cytokines in chronic heart failure: potential therapeutic implications. *Ann Med* 2005; **37**:74–85.

92 Stewart AL, Greenfield S, Hays RD, et al. Functional status and well-being of patients with chronic conditions – results from the medical outcomes study. *JAMA* 1989; **262**:907–913.

93 Fryback DG, Dasbach EJ, Klein R, et al. The Beaver Dam health outcomes study – initial catalog of health-state quality factors. *Med Dec Making* 1993; **13**:89–102.

94 Juenger J, Schellberg D, Kraemer S, et al. Health related quality of life in patients with congestive heart failure: comparison with other chronic diseases and relation to functional variables. *Heart* 2002; **87**:235–241.

95 Koenig HG. Depression in hospitalized older patients with congestive heart failure. *Gen Hosp Psych* 1998; **20**:29–43.

96 Levenson JW, McCarthy EP, Lynn J, et al. The last six months of life for patients with congestive heart failure. *J Am Geriatr Soc* 2000; **48**:S101–S109.

97 Krumholz HM, Phillips RS, Hamel MB, et al. Resuscitation preferences among patients with severe congestive heart failure: results from the SUPPORT project. *Circulation* 1998; **98**:648–655.

98 Krumholz HM, Phillips RS, Hamel MB, et al. Resuscitation preferences among patients with severe congestive heart failure: results from the SUPPORT project. *Circulation* 1998; **98**:648–655.

99 Murray SA, Boyd K, Kendall M, et al. Dying of lung cancer or cardiac failure: a community-based, prospective qualitative interview study of patients and their carers. *BMJ* 2002; **325**:931–34.

100 Haldeman GA, Croft JB, Giles WH, Rashidee A. Hospitalization of patients with heart failure: national hospital discharge survey 1985–1995. *Am Heart J* 1999; **137**:352–60.

101 Westert GP, Lagoe RJ, Keskimaki I, et al. An international study of hospital read-missions and related utilization in Europe and the USA. *Health Policy* 2002; **61**:269–278.

102 Stewart S, MacIntyre K, McCleod ME, et al. Trends in heart failure hospitalisations in Scotland, 1990–1996: an epidemic that has reached its peak? *Eur Heart J* 2001; **22**: 209–217.

103 MacIntyre K, Capewell S, Stewart S, et al. Evidence of improving prognosis in heart failure: trends in case-fatality in 66,547 patients hospitalised between 1986 and 1995. *Circulation* 2000; **102**:1126–1131.

104 Ho KKL, Anderson KM, Karmel WB, et al. Survival after the onset of congestive heart failure in the Framingham Heart Study subjects. *Circulation* 1993; **88**:107–115.

105 Stewart S, MacIntyre K, Hole DA, et al. More malignant than cancer? Five-year survival following a first admission for heart failure in Scotland? *Eur J Heart Failure* 2001; **3**:315–322.

106 Peeters A, Mamun AA, Willekens F, et al. for NEDCOM. A cardiovascular life history: a life course analysis of the original Framingham Heart Study cohort. *Eur Heart J* 2002; **23**:458–466.

107 Jong P, Vowineckel E, Liu PP, et al. Prognosis and determinants of survival in patients newly hospitalised for heart failure: a population based study. *Arch Intern Med* 2002; **162**:1689–1694.

108 Cowie MR, Wood DA, Coats AJS, et al. Survival of patients with a new diagnosis of heart failure: a population based study. *Heart* 2001; **83**:505–510.

109 Lynn J. An 88-year-old woman facing the end of life. *JAMA* 1997; **277**(20):1633–1640.

110 Brenna TD, Haas GJ. The role of prophylactic implantable cardioverter defibrillators in heart failure: recent trials usher in a new era of device therapy. *Curr Heart Fail Rep* 2005; **2**:40–45.

111 Levy D, Kenchaiah S, Larson MG, et al. Long-term trends in the incidence of and survival with heart failure. *N Engl J Med* 2002; **347**:1397–1402.

112 Jouven X, Desnos M, Guerot C, et al. Idiopathic atrial fibrillation as a risk factor for mortality. The Paris Prospective Study. *Eur Heart J* 1999; **20**:896–899.

113 Fuster V, Ryden LE, Asinger RW, et al. for the ACC, AHA, ESC & NASPE. ACC/AHA/ESC guidelines for the management of patients with atrial fibrillation. *Circulation* 2002; **104**:2118–2150.

114 Coumel P. Neural aspects of paroxysmal atrial fibrillation. In: Falk RH, Prodrid PJ,

eds. *Atrial Fibrillation: Mechanisms and Management.* New York: Raven Press, 1992, pp. 109–125.

115 Frost L, Johnsen SP, Pedersen L, et al. Seasonal variation in hospital discharge diagnosis of atrial fibrillation: a population-based study. *Epidemiology* 2002; **13**:211–215.

116 Murphy NF, Stewart S, MacIntyre K, et al. Seasonal variation in morbidity and mortality related to atrial fibrillation. *Int J Cardiol* 2004; **97**:283–288.

117 Wolf PA, Benjamin EJ, Belanger AJ, et al. Secular trends in the prevalence of atrial fibrillation: The Framingham Study. *Am Heart J* 1996; **131**:790–795.

118 Kannel WB, Wolf PA, Benjamin EJ, et al. Prevalence, incidence, prognosis, and predisposing conditions for atrial fibrillation: population-based estimates. *Am J Cardiol* 1998; **82**:2N–9N

119 Bharti S, Lev M. Histology of the normal and diseases atrium. In: Falk RH, Prodrid PJ, eds. *Atrial Fibrillation: Mechanisms and Management.* New York: Raven Press, 1992, pp. 15–39.

120 Moe GK, Abildskov JA. Atrial fibrillation as a self-sustaining arrhythmia independent of focal discharge. *Am Heart J* 1959; **58**:59–70.

121 Moe GK, Abildskov JA. Observations on the ventricular dysrhythmia associated with atrial fibrillation in the dog heart. *Circ Res* 1964; **4**:447–460.

122 Berry C, Stewart S, Payne EM, et al. Electrical cardioversion for atrial fibrillation: outcomes in 'real life' clinical practice. *Int J Cardiol* 2001; **81**:29–35.

123 Skanes AC, Mandapati R, Berenfeld O, et al. Spatiotemporal periodicity during atrial fibrillation in the isolated sheep heart. *Circulation* 1998; **98**:1236–1248.

124 Yue L, Feng J, Gaspo R, et al. Ionic remodeling underlying action potential changes in a canine model of atrial fibrillation. *Circ Res* 1997; **81**:512–525.

125 Manios EG, Kanoupakis EM, Mavrakis HE, et al. Sinus pacemaker function after cardioversion of chronic atrial fibrillation: is sinus node remodeling related with recurrence? *J Cardiovasc Electrophysiol* 2001; **12**:800–806.

126 Redfield MM, Kay GN, Jenkins LS, et al. Tachycardia-related cardiomyopathy a common cause of ventricular dysfunction in patients with atrial fibrillation referred for atrioventricular ablation. *Mayo Clin Proc* 2000; **75**:790–795.

127 Wolf P, Mitchell J, Baker C, et al. Impact of atrial fibrillation on mortality, stroke and medical costs. *Arch Intern Med* 1998; **158**:229–234.

128 Lip GY. The prothrombotic state in atrial fibrillation. New insights, more questions and clear answers needed. *Am Heart J* 2000; **140**:348–350.

129 Lip GY. Does atrial fibrillation confer a hypercoagulable state? Virchow's triad revisited. *J Am Coll Cardiol* 1999; **33**:1424–1426.

130 Stewart S, Hart CL, Hole DA, et al. A population-based study of the long-term risks associated with atrial fibrillation: 20-year follow-up of the Renfrew/Paisley Study. *Am J Med* 2002; **113**:359–364.

131 Juenger J, Schellberg D, Kraemer S, et al. Health related quality of life in patients with congestive heart failure: comparison with other chronic diseases and relation to functional variables. *Heart* 2002; **87**:235–241.

132 Stewart S, MacIntyre K, McCleod MC, et al. Trends in hospital activity, morbidity and case fatality related to atrial fibrillation in Scotland, 1986–1996. *Eur Heart J* 2001; **22**:693–701.

133 Frost L, Vestergaard P, Mosekilde L, et al. Trends in incidence and mortality in the hospital diagnosis of atrial fibrillation or flutter in Denmark, 1990–1999. *Int J Cardiol* 2005; **103**:78-84.

134 Stewart S, Murphy N, McGuire A, et al. The current cost of angina pectoris to the National Health Service in the United Kingdom. *Heart* 2003; **89**:848–853.

135 British Heart Foundation Coronary Heart Disease Statistics: http://www.bhf .org.uk/professionals/index.asp?secondlevel=519. Accessed June 2005.

136 American Heart Association – national and international statistics: http://www. americanheart.org/downloadable/heart/1105390918119HDSStats2005Update .pdf. Accessed June 2005.

137 McMurray JJV, Stewart S. The burden of heart failure. *Eur Heart J* 2003; **5**:I3–I113.

138 McDonagh TA, Morrison CE, Lawrence A, et al. Symptomatic and asymptomatic left-ventricular systolic dysfunction in an urban population. *Lancet* 1997; **350**: 829–833.

139 Davies M, Hobbs F, Davis R, et al. Prevalence of left ventricular systolic dysfunction and heart failure in the Echocardiographic Heart of England Screening Study: a population based study. *Lancet* 2001; **358**:439–444.

140 Mosterd A, Hoes AW, de Bruyne MC, et al. Prevalence of heart failure and left ventricular dysfunction in the general population: the Rotterdam Study. *Eur Heart J* 1999; **20**:447–455.

141 Schunkert H, Broeckel U, Hense HW, et al. Left ventricular dysfunction. *Lancet* 1998; **351**:372.

142 Gardin JM, Siscovick D, Anton-Culver H, et al. Sex, age and disease effect echocardiographic left ventricular mass and systolic function in the free-living elderly. The Cardiovascular Health Study. *Circulation* 1995; **91**:1739–1748.

143 Devereux RB, Roman MJ, Paranicas M, et al. A population based assessment of left ventricular systolic dysfunction in middle-aged and older adults: the Strong Heart Study. *Am Heart J* 2001; **141**:439–446.

144 Nielsen OW, Hilden J, Larsen CT, et al. Cross-sectional study estimating prevalence of heart failure and left ventricular systolic dysfunction in community patients at risk. *Heart* 2001; **86**:172–178.

145 Vasan RS, Larson MG, Benjamin EJ, et al. Congestive heart failure in subjects with normal versus reduced left ventricular ejection fraction: prevalence and mortality in a population-based cohort. *J Am Coll Cardiol* 1999; **33**:1948–1955.

146 Ceia F, Fonseca C, Mota T, et al. Prevalence of chronic heart failure in Southwestern Europe: the EPICA Study. *Eur J Heart Fail* 2002; **4**:531–539.

147 McMurray J, McDonagh T, Morrison CE, et al. Dargie HJ. Trends in hospitalization for heart failure in Scotland 1980–1990. *Eur Heart J* 1993; **14**:1158–1162.

148 Rodriguez-Artalejo F, Guallar-Castillon P, Banegas Banegas JR, et al. Trends in hospitalization and mortality for heart failure in Spain, 1980–1993. *Eur Heart J* 1997; **18**:1771–1779.

149 Abraham WT, Adams KF, Fonarow GC. In-hospital mortality in patients with acute decompensated heart failure requiring intravenous vasoactive medications: an analysis from the Acute Decompensated Heart Failure National Registry (ADHERE). *J Am Coll Cardiol* 2005; **46**:57–64.

150 Eriksson H, Wilhelmsen L, Caidahl K, et al. Epidemiology and prognosis of heart failure. *Z Kardiol* 1991; **80**:1–6.

151 Doughty R, Yee T, Sharpe N, et al. Hospital admissions and deaths due to congestive heart failure in New Zealand, 1988–91. *NZ Med J* 1995; **108**:473–475.

152 Reitsma JB, Mosterd A, de Craen AJM, et al. Increase in hospital admission rates for heart failure in The Netherlands, 1980–1993. *Heart* 1996; **76**:388–392.

153 Stewart S, MacIntyre K, McCleod ME, et al. Trends in heart failure hospitalisations in Scotland, 1990–1996:An epidemic that has reached its peak? *Eur Heart J* 2001; **22**:209–217.

154 Mosterd A, Reitsma JB, Grobbee DE. ACE inhibition and hospitalisation rates for heart failure in The Netherlands, 1980–1998. The end of an epidemic? *Heart* 2002; **87**:75–76.

155 Ng TP, Niti M. Trends and ethnic differences in hospital admissions and mortality for congestive heart failure in the elderly in Singapore, 1991 to 1998. *Heart* 2003; **89**:865–870.

156 Swedberg K, Köster M, Rosen M, et al. Decreasing one-year mortality from heart failure in Sweden: data from the Swedish Hospital Discharge Registry – 1988–2000. *J Am Coll Cardiol* 2002; **41**:190A.

157 Westert GP, Lagoe RJ, Keskimaki I, et al. An international study of hospital readmissions and related utilization in Europe and the USA. *Health Policy* 2002; **61**:269–278.

158 Murray J, Hart W, Rhodes G. An evaluation of the cost of heart failure to the National Health Service in the UK. *Br J Med Econ* 1993; **6**:91–98.

159 Stewart S, Jenkins A, Buchan S, et al. The current cost of heart failure in the UK: an economic analysis. *Eur J Heart Fail* 2002; **4**:361–371.

160 Kenchaiah S, Evans JC, Levy D, et al. Obesity and the risk of heart failure. *N Engl J Med* 2002; **347**(5):305–313.

161 Stewart S, MacIntyre K, Capewell S, McMurray JJV. An ageing population and heart failure: an increasing burden in the 21st century? *Heart.* 2003; **89**:49–53.

162 Kelly DT. Our future society: a global challenge. *Circulation* 1997; **95**:2459–2464.

163 Bonneux L, Barendregt JJ, Meeter K, et al. Estimating clinical morbidity due to ischaemic heart disease and congestive heart failure: the future rise of heart failure. *Am J Publ Health* 1994; **84**:20–28.

164 Feinberg WM, Blackshear JL, Laupacis A, et al. Prevalence, age distribution and gender of patients with atrial fibrillation: analysis and implications. *Arch Intern Med* 1995; **155**:469–473.

165 Stewart S, Murphy N, Walker A, et al. The cost of an emerging epidemic – an economic analysis of atrial fibrillation in the UK. *Heart* 2004; **90**:286–292.

166 Stewart S, Hart CL, Hole DA, et al. Population prevalence, incidence and predictors of atrial fibrillation in the Renfrew/Paisley Study. *Heart* 2001; **86**:516–521.

167 Wihelmsen L, Rosengren A, Lappas G. Hospitalizations for atrial fibrillation in the general male population: morbidity and risk factors. *J Intern Med* 2001; **250**:382–89.

168 Anonymous. Atrial fibrillation as a contributing cause of death and medicare hospitalization–United States, 1999. *MMWR Morb Mortal Wkly Rep* 2003; **52**:130–131.

169 Stewart S, MacIntyre K, McCleod MC, Bailey AE, McMurray JJV. Trends in hospital activity, morbidity and case fatality related to atrial fibrillation in Scotland, 1986–1996. *Eur Heart J* 2001; **22**:693–701.

170 Stewart S. Atrial fibrillation in the 21st Century: The new cardiac "Cinderella" and new horizons for cardiovascular nursing. *Eur J Cardiovasc Nursing* 2002; **2**:115–121.

171 Stewart S, McMurray JJV. Atrial fibrillation and the ageing population: an emerging epidemic? *Eur Heart J* 2002; **23**:617.

172 Youman P, Wilson K, Harraf F, et al. The economic burden of stroke in the United Kingdom. *Pharmacoeconomics* 2003; **21**:43–50.

173 Hravnak M, Hoffman LA, Saul MI, et al. Resource utilization related to atrial fibrillation after coronary artery bypass grafting. *Am J Crit Care* 2002; **11**:228–238.

174 Maier W, Windecker S, Boersma E, et al. Evolution of percutaneous transluminal coronary angioplasty in Europe (1992 – 1996). *Eur Heart J* 2001; **22**:1733–1740.

175 Stewart S, Blue L, Walker A, et al. An economic analysis of specialist heart failure management in the UK – can we afford not to implement it? *Eur Heart J* 2002; **23**:1369–1378.

176 Tinetti ME, Bogardus ST, Agostini JV. Potential pitfalls of disease-specific guidelines for patients with multiple conditions. *N Engl J Med* 2004; **351**(27):2870–2874.

177 Horowitz JD, Sia STB, Macdonald PS, et al. Perhexiline maleate treatment for severe angina pectoris- correlations with pharmacokinetics. *Int J Cardiol* 1986; **13**:219–229.

178 Kennedy JA, Unger SA, Horowitz JD. Inhibition of Carnitine Palmitoyltransferase-1 in rat heart and liver by perhexiline and amiodarone. *Biochem Pharmacol* 1996; **52**:273–280.

179 Lee L, Horowitz JD, Frenneaux M. Metabolic manipulation in ischaemic heart disease, a novel approach to treatment. *Eur Heart J* 2004; **25**:634–641.

180 Gupta R, Tang WH, Young JB. Patterns of beta-blocker utilization in patients with chronic heart failure: experience from a specialized outpatient heart failure clinic. *Am Heart J* 2004; **147**:79–83.

181 Zimetbaum P, Reynolds MR, Ho KK, et al. Impact of a practice guideline for patients with atrial fibrillation on medical resource utilization and costs. *Am J Cardiol* 2003; **92**:677–681.

Section 2
Effective Models of Chronic Cardiac Care

CHAPTER 3

Slowing the progression of cardiovascular disease: innovative approaches to cardiac rehabilitation and secondary prevention

3.1 Introduction

As noted in the previous section of this book, chronic cardiac disease represents a growing epidemic in ageing populations that requires a systematic approach to proactively address "secondary prevention" (i.e. minimizing *future* morbid and prematurely fatal events due to disease progression) and improving the *current* management of the disease to immediately improve quality of life and reduce the probability of acute crises. It is within this context that cardiac rehabilitation (in this chapter it will be abbreviated to CR) programs are ideally positioned to play a pivotal role in the provision of many of the components of comprehensive CVD risk-reduction services [1]. The World Health Organization (WHO) defines CR as:

> "the sum of activities required to ensure cardiac patients the best possible physical, mental and social conditions so that they may, by their own efforts, resume and maintain as normal a place as possible in the community"[2].

Since this early definition there have been a number of revisions, and CR has also evolved to include secondary prevention as a core component (i.e. stabilizing, slowing or even reversing the underlying atherosclerotic process) as well as optimizing a patient's physical and psychosocial functioning following an acute event (post AMI)[3].

The traditional and most researched model of CR consists of clients and their partners attending a group outpatient program conducted by a multi-disciplinary team commonly involving nurses, medical staff, dieticians, physiotherapists, and social workers. Services are provided for a period of four to 12 weeks and are predominantly based in outpatient hospital settings.

Programs include supervised physical activity, risk factor education, advice on psychological and social functioning, and referral to maintenance CR services if available [4]. The clinical benefits of traditional CR have been demonstrated in several publications including meta-analyses and a Cochrane review [3,5–9]. These benefits include improvements in the following parameters:

- Physical and psychosocial functioning
- Improvements in coronary risk factor profiles
- Reduced smoking rates
- Decreased rates of subsequent coronary events
- Reduced hospitalization, and
- A 26% reduction in cardiac mortality during active follow-up* [5,7–9].

However, the extent to which traditional CR programs can successfully deliver the services necessary for comprehensive cardiovascular disease risk reduction is currently limited by several fundamental deficiencies [1]. These fundamental deficiencies result in an internationally observed low uptake rate for CR. It was suggested that this low uptake can be explained by CR service-, patient-, and social/environmental-related barriers to participation in CR [10,11]. This chapter discusses these barriers to participation in CR as well as innovative approaches to overcoming the barriers to improve access and availability of CR.

3.2 Barriers to participation in cardiac rehabilitation

Service-related factors predictive of low-uptake of CR include the lack of availability and accessibility of a program, as well as a lack of program capacity to enroll referred participants or provide the necessary flexibility to maximize participation; a lack of referral to the program; and the strength of a physician's recommendation to attend [11–15]. Accessibility or travel distance is a particular deterrent for urban populations, and is even more problematic for people living in rural and remote areas [11]. Patient-related factors predictive of low-uptake of CR include: advancing age; female gender (women and the elderly often report that they feel out of place in CR programs); poor functional capacity; beliefs that their illness could be cured rather than controlled; low self efficacy and self esteem; and lack of motivation to participate [11,16,17]. Social/environmental-related barriers to participation in CR include: low socioeconomic status; low education level; lack of family support; work or time constraints; and lack of transport [11,13,18].

Figure 3.1 is a model of reported CR service-, patient- and social or environmental-related barriers to participation in CR, and highlights the fact that there is overlap between the classification of these barriers as patient-, service-, or social/environmental-related. For example, whilst age may predict lower CR participation, the actual causes of this pattern may be complex and

---

*It is important to remember that there is no "cure" for coronary artery disease, most treatments can be regarded as palliative, and slowing the progression of the underlying disease process is the major therapeutic goal.

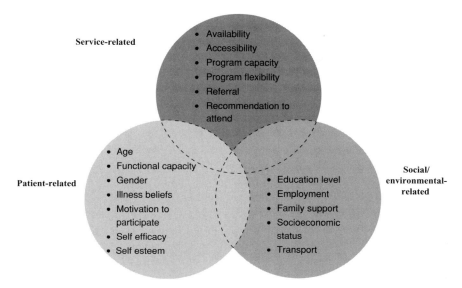

Figure 3.1 A model of barriers to participation in cardiac rehabilitation program: lessons for chronic cardiac care.

related to limited program capacity, flexibility, or resources to allow for older patients [19]. In addition, lack of transport is commonly reported as a barrier to participation in CR. However, beneath this barrier there is a complex web of cost-benefit calculations, patient values, and perceptions [20].

The dropout rates the dropout rates from exercise programs among those who do attend traditional CR range from 20% in the first three months, to 50% at six to 12 months [21]. Dropout rates have been reported to be greater in high intensity exercise programs and those that are *poorly organized*. Smokers, patients who have had more than one AMI [21,22] and women are more likely to drop out [23]. Dropout has been shown to be related to patients' confusion about the aims, content, and structure of rehabilitation programs, their own beliefs, or the information given by health professionals about the seriousness of their heart condition [24,25]. As a result of these service-, patient-, environmental or social-related barriers to participation and adherence, CR services are underutilized and there is a substantial treatment gap. Although reported CR program participant rates very from country to country, overall, it is estimated that only 10–30% of eligible patients participate in CR programs in Western developed countries.

Clearly the treatment gap in CR participation remains a frustrating impediment to fulfilling the potential for improving quality of life and longevity through cardiovascular disease risk-reduction interventions [31]. Hence there is a need to bridge the treatment gap by developing innovative or alternative approaches to CR that would provide everyone with, or at risk of, cardiovascular disease access to comprehensive, high quality, and affordable risk-reduction interventions that would be appropriate for their specific needs [1].

3.3 Alternative models of cardiac rehabilitation

Much of the work in alternative approaches to CR since the 1980s has been conducted by researchers of Stanford University, California, United States [32]. The alternative models of primary and secondary prevention pioneered at Stanford include home-based CR [33], and the lifestyle approach for coronary risk factor modification [33]. More recently, a number of innovative home-based CR programs have used the Internet as a method for patient communication and education [10,34,35].

Home-based cardiac rehabilitation

Home-based CR programs were first developed to overcome some of the patient-, social or environmental-, and service-related barriers to participation in traditional CR, that have been outlined above. Debusk and colleagues from Stanford were the first to show the feasibility of home-based exercise training in enhancing the functional capacity of uncomplicated post-MI patients in the 1980s [36]. They used trans-telephonic ECG monitoring to enhance the safety of the home-based training, and the improvement in functional capacity at six months postevent among patients exercising in a home environment was similar to that of patients exercising in a medically supervised program. The cost of this equally effective intervention was also one-half that of a traditional CR program (US$328 vs $720 per patient per year in 1985) Several well designed studies have since demonstrated that home-based programs can be safe and effective for patients following a cardiac events [27,33–35,37–48], and the key studies have been outlined below.

In the 1990s, Debusk and colleagues developed and studied a physician-directed, nurse-managed, home-based care management system for coronary risk factor intervention [33]. Specially trained nurses (care-managers) initiated interventions for smoking cessation, exercise training, and diet/medication treatment for hyperlipidemia. Nurses spent approximately *nine hours* with patients over a 12-month period. Intervention postdischarge was primarily by telephone and mail. By 12 months, this care-management approach resulted in significantly better outcomes for functional ability, cholesterol levels, and smoking rates. In addition, the intervention resulted in higher compliance rates for cholesterol and blood pressure medication use, exercise, and smoking cessation than is typically observed in traditional CR programs. The positive results of this trial lead the investigators to develop a clinical program called MULTIFIT that was available for use by organizations. The average yearly cost per patient of the MULTIFIT program was US$541 compared with $2200 for a traditional CR program [32,49].

Around the same time, Haskell and colleagues, also of Stanford University, were developing the Stanford Coronary Risk Intervention Project (SCRIP) [40]. The intervention group received an individualized home-based program from a SCRIP nurse involving a low-fat and low-cholesterol diet, exercise, weight loss, smoking cessation, and medications to favorable lower lipoprotein profiles. Subjects were supported by telephone and mail, returning every two to three months to the clinic throughout a four-year period. The SCRIP program resulted in highly significant improvements in cholesterol levels, exercise capacity, and intake of dietary fat and cholesterol when compared with the control group. The SCRIP program was also shown to favorably alter the rate of luminal narrowing of coronary arteries of men and women with coronary artery disease, as well as decrease hospitalizations for clinical cardiac events.

In the 1990s in the United Kingdom, Lewin and colleagues developed a home-based program that included a patient resource called the "Heart Manual" [38]. This resource included a six-week education program with a relaxation and stress management tape. Subjects followed the resource with the assistance of a facilitator who gave subjects general advice (for approximately 10 minutes) via the telephone, home visit, or in the clinic at one, three, and six weeks postenrolment. Compared with the control group, the intervention group at six weeks had significantly lower anxiety, depression, and better general health; at six months had significantly fewer GP/primary care visits, hospital readmissions, and better general health; at 12 months had significantly lower anxiety, GP visits, and better general health. The original trial results have since been reproduced [50–53], and the Heart Manual approach has now been adopted by more than 200 provider organizations in the UK [53].

In 2000, Ades and colleagues [42] conducted a multicenter trial to compare the effectiveness of home-based, transtelephonically monitored CR with traditional CR [42]. The effects of a home-based, three-month, transtelephonically monitored rehabilitation program with simultaneous voice and electrocardiographic transmission to a centrally located nurse coordinator were compared with the effects of a standard on-site rehabilitation program. The results indicated that quality of life and peak aerobic capacity improved to a similar degree in the two groups, and there were no exercise-related medical events in more than 3000 hours of exercise training in either group [42].

In recent years, Vale and colleagues [45] developed a home-based program to encourage patients to reach target levels of coronary heart disease risk factors (The COACH Program) in Australia. Cardiac patients were recruited in hospital then contacted by telephone five times over a six-month period. Patients were coached to work with their physician to achieve the target levels for their total cholesterol as well as other risk factors for coronary heart disease. At six months follow-up, the intervention group achieved a significantly greater improvement in: cholesterol (total and LDL); blood pressure; weight loss; fat, cholesterol, and fiber intake; anxiety (assessed with State-Trait Anxiety Inventory); physical activity; self-perception of quality of life; and cardiac symptoms. The dropout rate for this program was 14%.

Internet-based models of cardiac rehabilitation

Some of the more recent alternative models to CR have included Internet-based programs [10,35]. Gordon and colleagues [34] developed a comprehensive cardiovascular disease risk reduction program for use in primary and secondary prevention settings (INTER$_x$VENT). The program was administered in clinical and community-based settings including: CR programs; hospitals; physician practices; work sites; shopping malls; health clubs; as well as from a call center using the Internet and telephone. Program staff used a computerized participant management and tracking system, and the intervention was based on several behavior change models, including social learning theory, stages of change model, and single concept learning theory. Typically the program was administered by nonphysician health care professionals whose services were integrated with the care provided by the participants' physicians. When administered by an exercise physiologist to low or moderate-risk coronary artery disease patients in a nonmedical setting, INTER$_x$VENT was at least as effective as facility-based CR and a physician supervised case-managed program [34].

In 2003, Southard and colleagues published the Heartlinks program, which was a case management system for the secondary prevention of coronary heart disease using the Internet as the primary link between a case manager and the patient, as well as their family members [35]. The case manager provided risk factor management support, education, and monitoring services to patients with cardiovascular disease. There were also separate interfaces for other health care providers including patient's physicians, dietitians, and psychologists. The patients accessed the program at their own pace and the program was customized on the basis of patients' risk factors and other demographic variables. The case manager interacted with the same patient electronically via secure communication lines, and the program facilitated the development of a supportive online community of patients with cardiovascular disease and their families through discussions groups and voluntary E-mail exchange. The results of a trial for patients with cardiovascular disease indicated that at six months, compared with usual care, fewer cardiovascular events and more weight loss occurred in the intervention group (resulting in a gross cost saving of US$1418 per patient). Whilst the differences between the groups in terms of blood pressure, lipid levels, depression scores, physical activity, and dietary habits were not statistically significant. The projected cost of the program per patient was US$453. The authors state that the program could be used as a stand alone cost-effective intervention for patients with cardiovascular disease, or in conjunction with traditional CR.

On the whole, alternative approaches to CR have been shown to be clinically effective and (in some cases) shown to reduce costs. The literature has shown that home-based CR using other forms of health professional-consumer contact besides the traditional group clinic-based session can be incorporated into CR or patient care, and can be used as: an adjunctive therapeutic modality, a method to extend the time frame of therapeutic contact, and an alternative when in-person contact is not possible or preferable [10,35,54]. A review of the literature does not clearly indicate which alternative approach to CR is the most effective, or the most appropriate medium or frequency of health professional-patient contact. However, in general the literature on alternative models of CR suggests that successful programs have included a number of common features. These features have included: individualized patient management (case or care management) and flexible health professional-consumer contact (clinic visits, home visits, telephone support, Internet support, and personal digital assistants); a level of risk stratification to ensure patients receive the most appropriate form of health professional-consumer contact; and consumers have generally received a consumer-focussed resource/s to direct them through the program (paper-based, audio tapes, video tapes, DVDs, or Internet-based information). These common features are discussed below.

3.4 Care management

Generically, care management is a process of planning, providing, and monitoring care of a designated group of patients over an extended period of time. Care management aims to provide quality health care along a continuum, to enhance the client's quality of life, and to control costs [55]. The single function that most distinguishes care management from other health care delivery approaches is centralized coordination of all aspects of care by one professional [56].

In CR, the care manager coordinates the patients' health care, although care management also emphasizes the active involvement of three parties: the patient, the family, and the multidisciplinary health team (see Table 3.1 [56]). In a pure care management model, the care manager-patient contact would begin at the time of diagnosis or hospital admission, continue through

Table 3.1 The three parties involved in care management in cardiac rehabilitation [56].

The patient	Personal responsibility is promoted through interactive participation, encouragement, and education. Patients receive "home work" to complete, tasks to perform (such as recording risk factor behavior logs and charts), and are requested to participate in completing their care plan [56]. Coaching is an effective technique that may empower and encourage the patient to set goals to make the necessary or desired behavior changes [57].
The family	The family is included as strong and consistent family support increases the likelihood of successful lifestyle change. Family members are invited to observe exercise sessions in action, to attend group classes, to participate in behavior changes with their loved ones, and to meet with the care manager for private discussions as required [56].
The multidisciplinary health team	The care manager is responsible for identifying and coordinating the needs of each patient to ensure that their problems are addressed effectively and expeditiously. Referral to other health professionals provides patients with the best available expertise to meet their rehabilitation needs [56].

treatment or recovery and rehabilitation, and most importantly follow the patient for an extended period of time (one to two years).

Care management can provide the external structure through which alternative models of CR are delivered as outlined above. Alternatively, care-management can be internally applied as the method of practice within an existing traditional CR program. For these programs, the care manager would be based at the hospital or in the community, and the newest functions would include the use of care plans and protocols, the focus on outcomes, and the integration of care across the health care continuum. When appropriately used in hospital settings, care management has been shown to effectively produce individual outcomes that contribute to risk reduction and an overall improvement in the effectiveness of the CR program [56]. Thus, existing traditional CR programs seeking to redesign their delivery mechanisms may wish to implement or extend a care management approach: components of which may already be in place, but under-utilized.

3.5 Risk stratification

It is well established that medically supervised, physician-directed, CR exercise programs that follow the guidelines are relatively safe. The occurrence of major cardiovascular events during supervised exercise in contemporary programs ranges from 1/50,000 to 1/120,000 patient-hours of exercise, with only two fatalities reported per 1.5 million patient-hours of exercise [58]. However, with the development of home-based CR programs, contemporary risk-stratification procedures for the management of coronary heart disease will help to identify patients who are at increased risk for exercise-related cardiovascular events, and who may require more intensive cardiac monitoring during exercise [26]. As a patient is referred to a CR program, the care manager should conduct an intake assessment, collaborating with other care providers to determine the most appropriate rehabilitation placement and program. In determining the most appropriate program for the patient, the care manager would need to consider the safety of the recommended physical activity program and the required level of supervision (i.e. risk stratification). Patients at high risk may require supervision during physical activity sessions, whilst moderate- to low- risk patients would require less frequent supervision or may be suitable for unsupervised exercise. In the present economic environment, CR programs need to be resource-sparing as they struggle to meet the demand of all eligible patients. Thus appropriate risk stratification may aid in the management of limited CR resources [59].

3.6 Educational strategies and resources in cardiac rehabilitation

Patient education is identified as an important component of disease management programs including CR, but the most effective educational strategies are not well defined [60]. The provision of educational information is not synonymous with patient education, and the provision of information alone is likely to be of limited benefit [61]. Verbal communication with health professionals remains the preferred method of information exchange, but patients prefer interactive multimedia technology such as computers and the Internet, as well as DVDs and videos, over simple written information [61]. In addition, the development of patient materials that support patient participation, decision making, and empowerment are recommended, and are also likely to be of greater benefit than the provision of information alone [61,62].

Decisional role preferences during health professional-patient interactions vary between patients and may vary over time. Most patients prefer a collaborative approach, whilst some people prefer an active role, and others, a more passive role. Patients preferring an active role need more detailed information, and there are a range of available options including materials that support patient participation during consultation, decision-aids, tailored personal communication, and consultation records. In particular, decision aids or shared decision making programs have been developed as adjuncts to counseling from practitioners. Decision aids improve knowledge, reduce decisional conflict, and stimulate patients to be more active in decision making without increasing their anxiety [62]. The shared decision making model has been advocated as a way of promoting clinical effectiveness [63]. This model differs from the informed choice model where the emphasis is on the patient to make the decisions, and the more traditional or biomedical model where the health professional makes the decisions [64]. Nevertheless, the patient's desire to participate will differ between patients and may differ within patients over time, so a variety of strategies and resources will be required to meet the needs of the target group. In all cases, the target group should be considered in planning and development to ensure that the materials are appropriate for them. It is also important to consider that not all components of a comprehensive CR program will be relevant to the patient (e.g. smoking cessation advice may be irrelevant for nonsmokers) and thus a CR program should be tailored to the patients' needs to maximize patient interest.

3.7 Beyond outpatient cardiac rehabilitation or secondary prevention programs – the ongoing management of coronary heart disease

As discussed previously, the management of the most common chronic conditions, chronic angina pectoris, CHF, and AF, is a complex process that requires the dedication of the patient, the patient's family, and a supportive and functional team of health professionals, or health system, over an extended period of time. Furthermore, the advancing age of patients with chronic cardiac disease adds to the complexity of ongoing management. However, CR programs do not continue for an extended period of time, and are commonly four to 12 weeks long only, relying on short-term exposure to lifestyle behaviors (exercise, diet, smoking cessation, and stress reduction) and risk factor modification to result in long-term improvements to quality of life and reduced morbidity and mortality. It is hoped that participants will maintain lifestyle changes and continue to undergo risk factor modification [65]. Unfortunately, several studies indicate that after completion of CR, exercise adherence greatly decreases, body weight increases, and serum lipid values *deteriorate* [66,67]. Thus some CR and secondary prevention programs have been designed to address the maintenance of lifestyle changes and risk factor modification following the completion of traditional CR programs [46,59,68,65].

Brubaker et al. developed a nine-month home-based exercise program to enable patients to maintain/improve their blood lipids, body composition, and functional capacity after exiting CR [46]. Patients exiting an initial traditional three-month CR program were assigned randomly to the home-based intervention (one home visit followed by weekly telephone calls and exercise logs) or usual care. A third group, randomly selected from patients who elected to remain in the traditional CR program for the same duration, was also examined. There were equally significant increases in metabolic equivalents and high-density lipoprotein, in all three groups, over time, indicating that the home-based CR program was as effective as the traditional program at improving/maintaining functional capacity, blood lipids, and body weight/composition. The authors suggested that the similar success of the usual care group was likely due to their prior experience in CR and knowledge of follow-up testing [46].

Lear et al. developed a multifactorial intervention aimed at the prevention of behavioral recidivism and risk factor deterioration following CR (Extensive Lifestyle Management Intervention Trial or ELMI) [65]. They investigated a randomized one-year multifactorial risk factor and lifestyle intervention in men and women with heart disease following CR. Intervention patients received exercise sessions, telephone follow-ups, and risk factor and lifestyle counseling. They found that adherence to the ELMI was high and, compared with usual care, there was a nonsignificant trend in favor of the ELMI for both the Framingham and Procam absolute risk scores [65].

While short-term participation in traditional CR programs usually results in numerous positive health changes as outlined above, compliance with longer-term behavior change following the completion of traditional CR programs is disappointingly *low*. Maintenance CR programs have been developed to enhance long-term adherence to healthy lifestyle behaviors; however, overall these studies have unfortunately had mixed results [46,59,65,68]. However, the lessons learned from the active management of traditional risk factors, should be integrated into the type of chronic cardiac disease management programs outlined in Chapter 4.

3.8 Summary

In summary, there is strong evidence to demonstrate the effectiveness of traditional cardiac rehabilitation (CR) programs. However, there is a significant treatment gap as a result of CR service-, patient-, and social or environmental-related barriers to participation. Since the 1980s, a number of innovative or alternative models of CR have been developed to overcome these barriers, and these models have largely been clinically effective, and in some cases cost-effective as well. Lessons learned from these innovative approaches to CR suggest that future models of CR would risk-stratify patients to ensure patients at high risk received more intensive care, whilst those at moderate or low risk would receive less frequent contact and rely more on community resources. The CR program would be individualized for the patient (care management), and consideration would be given to the preferred mode of service delivery (such as a dedicated clinic, via the telephone, internet or personal digital assistant, or another means of delivered care) for the particular target group, and acknowledgement that the preferred or most appropriate mode of service delivery may change during the course of the CR program. Finally, health professionals involved in CR would consider the extent to which the patient wished to be involved in a shared decision-making model, and all patient materials would be appropriate for the target population.

All of the lessons learned in relation to the practical application of CR, based on the key issues relating to the following, should be considered in relation to the practical management of chronic cardiac disease:

- The overall effectiveness of targeting cardiovascular risk factors to prevent disease progression.
- The need for delineation of risk and "titration" of prevention based on the same.
- The problems of accessibility and the subsequent need to offer "innovative" modes of delivery (e.g. interactive technology).
- The clear need to consider the individual beliefs and needs of the patient (more fully explored in Chapter 6).

Finally, given that behavioral recidivism and risk factor deterioration is common following the completion of traditional CR programs, and that many individuals in whom such a phenomenon has occurred will develop chronic cardiac disease and therefore require chronic cardiac care. This demands consideration of the factors that have "led" each patient to develop chronic cardiac disease (i.e. failure of primary and secondary prevention to date), and strategic attempts to make a substantial difference in this regard. It is within this context that the following chapter explores the relative success of nurse-led, CHF management programs.

CHAPTER 4

Chronic CHF management programs: an exemplar for chronic cardiac care

4.1 Introduction

As indicated in the previous chapter in relation to secondary prevention, although it is often easy to first identify a problem and then identify what needs to be done to address such a problem, it is more than likely that implementing so-called "solutions" in health will fail to meet initial expectations; particularly when one considers that it requires the complexities and demands of an unwieldy health care system to satisfy and agree with the complexities of human thinking and behavior!

It is within this context that one of the most successful "therapeutic advances" in modern-day health care has emerged to defy traditional expectations of another "failed" initiative. As described in this chapter, predominantly, nurse-led CHF management programs (abbreviated to CHF-MPs in this chapter) have no doubt considered the relative merits (and weaknesses) of cardiac rehabilitation and other forms of "secondary prevention" to tackle the enormous complexities and issues surrounding the effective management of CHF. Overall, CHF-MPs appear to be winning the battle (remembering that without a cure there is no "absolute" win other than improving the lives and deaths of patients to the greatest possible extent) and are beginning to contribute to improved CHF-related outcomes at the population level. The potential parallels for similar improvements in other forms of chronic cardiac disease (particularly given that they often form part of the syndrome of CHF) are obvious. As such, this chapter outlines the key characteristics and evidence in favor of this form of intervention.

4.2 Key issues that have influenced the development of CHF-MPs

Apart from the obvious and increasing pressure imposed by CHF in nearly all developed countries, predicating the development of more effective health care programs, a range of issues have influenced the purpose, structure, and complexity of modern-day CHF-MPs:

- It is clear that apart from preventing "at risk" individual patients from ultimately developing CHF (obviously established primary prevention strategies [69] and, more recently, the HOPE Study [70] are relevant to this) and applying the type of "secondary prevention" programs of care outlined in Chapter 3, the greatest cost-benefits are likely to be derived from targeting those who have already* been hospitalized with CHF – particularly old and fragile patients at high risk of subsequent morbidity and mortality.
- It is important to recognize that whilst a significant proportion of CHF-related admissions are indeed avoidable, a sizable proportion is likely to be either inevitable for adequate treatment of an acute clinical crisis, or desirable to provide for adequate investigation and future management: particularly if it is their first acute presentation.
- Precipitating factors leading to a CHF-related admission are often multifactorial and interrelated. The typical profile of the older patient with CHF who has been hospitalized (e.g. with acute decompensated CHF secondary to uncontrolled AF and underlying anaemia) is often complex and identifying contributory factors is often nebulous.
- Given the often extensive list of concurrent disease states in older patients with CHF, it is often difficult to determine its exact role in precipitating acute events. As such, the proportion of hospitalizations that can be identified as directly attributable to the syndrome (even if frequent) is often less than 50%.
- Regardless of the purpose of an intervention designed to limit CHF-related morbidity rates (and therefore costs), and the often overwhelming imperative to minimize the expense of a program whilst maximizing subsequent cost savings, it is important to appreciate the degree of comfort and satisfaction patients with CHF derive from receiving individualized care and support.

Given the above, it should come as no surprise how the general body of research in this area has developed and the general direction it has taken. Most of the early studies (between 1995 and 2000) testing the relative benefits of programs of care in CHF-targeted hospitalized patients and applied interventions during or immediately following their index admission. Not surprisingly, those studies targeting typically older "high risk" patients have proven to be the most cost-effective when resulting in reduced hospital admissions and associated stay in the presence of high underlying morbidity and mortality rates.

Studies to date have typically worked on the assumption that an approximate halving in recurrent hospitalization in the short- to medium-term is feasible. Although there has been a trend toward a more specific and exclusive

---

*For a more detailed and specific description of CHF management refer to Stewart S, Blue L (eds). *Improving outcomes in chronic CHF: specialist nurse intervention from research to practice.* London: BMJ Books, 2004.

focus on managing CHF more effectively, the greatest cost-benefits have been derived from those programs of care that reduce "all-cause" readmissions (e.g. by focusing on general treatment adherence issues) rather than CHF-related readmissions alone. Related to the cost-dynamics of applying an additional component of health care in order to subsequently reduce costs, there was an obvious need to apply a relatively "cheap" but effective intervention, (i.e. which reduces all-cause recurrent stay). Given the complex nature of CHF and factors precipitating clinical instability, it was perhaps not surprising that one-dimensional interventions (e.g. providing pre-discharge education) have proved to be relatively ineffective and were quickly discarded in favor of flexible but individualized interventions delivered or coordinated (with a multidisciplinary context) by suitably trained nurses.

Over a relatively short period of time the role of the "specialist CHF nurse" (or other derivatives) has expanded to maximize the time they can spend with the patient – most notably prescribing and titration of pharmacotherapy (e.g. ACE inhibitors, beta-blockers, and latterly spironolactone and angiotensin receptor blockers). Given the inherent satisfaction of CHF patients with this type of contact (i.e. with a caring nurse), and the emergence of academic nurses as principal investigators of these studies, it should come as no surprise that spending time with patients on a individual basis has become an important feature of these programs. In order to "protect" this individual time from future cost-cutting measures, it will be important for specialist CHF nurses to quantify the therapeutic benefits of such contact.

It is within this context that the number of postdischarge, CHF programs of care involving a key role for the specialist nurses has exploded. A number of key features are common to nearly all these programs:
- A multidisciplinary approach.
- Individualized care.
- Patient education and counseling (often involving the family/carer).
- Intensive follow-up to detect and address clinical problems on a proactive basis.
- Strategies to both apply evidence-based pharmacological treatment and improve adherence.
- Application of nonpharmacological strategies where appropriate (e.g. fluid and electrolyte management and exercise programs).
- Patient-initiated access to appropriate advice and support [71].

As will be discussed in more detail in Chapter 6, a major goal of this type of program is to encourage a greater level of effective self-care behaviors in the majority of patients (e.g. daily weight monitoring, applying a diuretic regimen, and recognizing signs of acute CHF and seeking appropriate health care) and only filling the "gaps" in certain cases (e.g. an older patient who lives alone). Determining the most desirable and effective role of interactive technology that is able to provide a greater level of patient surveillance (e.g. via computerized tracking of a patient's clinical status using a home monitoring device) while encouraging a degree of independence from the health care system is probably yet to be determined. Certainly, as will be described in a separate section later in this Chapter, there is a growing body of research examining the role of "remote" health care and striking the balance between providing therapeutic human contact, promoting self-care behaviors and monitoring a patient's clinical status without creating a "Big Brother" scenario of excessive intrusion, is a major challenge in the future.

4.3 The evidence in support of nurse-led programs of care in CHF

There now exists an increasing body of research to support the application of postdischarge, CHF-MPs with a major role for a specialist CHF nurse in most cases – the one exception being a pharmacist-based intervention [72]. However, it is important to note that a large number of published research studies have either involved a small number of patients, have had limited follow-up, or measured the influence of a particular program using pre- and post-testing periods or historical control data. While such studies are important to the general body of literature, it is most appropriate to examine the results of appropriately powered studies that employed a randomized design – particularly as other designs inherently inflate the observed magnitude of effect. Two "landmark" studies played an important part in the development and application of CHF-MPs.

Rich and colleagues (1995)

In the first properly powered and conducted study of its type, Rich [73] found that a nurse-led, multidisciplinary intervention (which involved a component of home visits) had beneficial effects as regards rates of hospital readmission, quality of life, and cost of care, within 90 days of discharge among "high risk" chronic CHF patients. The intervention consisted of comprehensive education of the patient and family, a prescribed diet, social service consultation, and planning for an early discharge, optimization of pharmacotherapy, and intensive home- and clinic-based follow-up with frequent telephone contact. At 90 days, survival without readmission was achieved in 91 of 142 (64%) intervention patients compared to 75 of 140 (54%) control patients ($P = 0.09$). There were 94 versus 53 readmissions in the control and intervention groups respectively ($P = 0.02$). These readmissions equated to a total of 865 versus 556 days of hospitalization (a 36% reduction) or 6.2 versus 3.9 days per patient ($P = 0.04$) [73].

Stewart and colleagues (1999–2005)

Following posthoc analyses of a large-scale randomized controlled study of chronically ill patients with a mixture of cardiac and noncardiac disease states [74], which showed that a nurse-led, multidisciplinary, home-based intervention was most effective in CHF [75,76], Stewart et al. prospectively examined a more HF-specific form of a nurse-led, home-based intervention in

200 patients (100 in each group) [77]. During six months follow-up the primary endpoint occurred more frequently in the usual care group (129 vs 77 primary events; $P = 0.02$). More intervention patients remained event-free (38 vs 51; $P = 0.04$). Overall, there were fewer unplanned readmissions (68 vs 118; $P = 0.03$) and associated days of hospitalization (460 vs 1173; $P = 0.02$) among patients assigned to the study intervention [77].

   The ultimate aim, of course, is reduced health care costs over the typical lifespan of the target patient cohort. For example, with the exception of the 10-year follow-up of the original CONSENSUS Study cohort [78], there are very few studies to suggest that clinically effective treatments in HF (including beta-blockers and spironolactone) are associated with sustained cost-benefits – particularly when such treatments are associated with prolonged survival and therefore the opportunity for further morbidity. With this major caveat in mind, Stewart and colleagues [79] recently examined the longer-term effects of the nurse-led, multidisciplinary, and home-based intervention on the 298 Australian patients participating in two of the randomized studies outlined above [76,77]. Median study follow-up was for 4.2 years and ranged from three to six years postdischarge. During prolonged follow-up, nearly all patients were either hospitalized or died. A total of 96 of 148 patients (65%) in the usual care group died. In comparison, a total of 83 of 149 patients (56%) subject to the study intervention had died and it was independently associated with a 28% relative risk reduction in mortality ($P < 0.05$). Despite the more prolonged survival in the study group (equivalent to an additional 817 months of survival overall) initially observed benefits in respect to recurrent hospital stay persisted over the longer-term. Moreover, although the relative difference in recurrent stay fell from approximately 60% at six months to 22% at three years with health care costs remaining substantially lower in the longer-term [79].

   Further follow-up of the same cohort at five years post intervention, indicated a total of 121 of 148 patients (82%) had died over the five years. In comparison to the initial 149 patients subject to home-based intervention, 92 had died (62%) (see Figure 4.1) [80]. Not only had the usual care group experienced greater mortality than the home-based intervention group at the five-year mark, but the number of unplanned admissions between the groups also varied. Of the 148 usual care patients, there were 507 unplanned admissions over the five years, compared to 444 unplanned admissions for those 149 patients enrolled in the home-based intervention. The costs related to these unplanned hospital admissions for both the home-based intervention and usual care groups was calculated to be AUD $1.86 million versus AUD $2.93 million, respectively. The interim cost-benefit ratio of better CHF management was demonstrated by the prolonged survival and lower unplanned admissions for the group, which represented a gain of 63 additional life-years and savings of AUD $81,000 per 100 patients treated – (see Figure 4.2) [80]. These findings demonstrate that CHF management programs not only improve survival, but are also highly likely to be cost-effective when systematically applied.

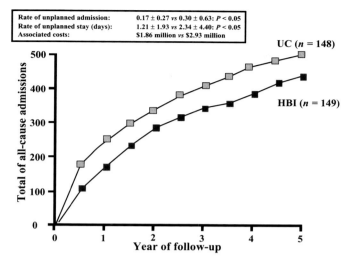

Figure 4.1 Five-year morbidity in CHF patients subject to home-based intervention versus usual postdischarge care [80].

Evidence from meta-analyses

In a recent systematic review and meta-analysis of 29 trials involving over 5000 patients with CHF randomized to a dedicated management program or usual postdischarge care, we found that overall, patients exposed to the intervention arms of these studies were significantly less likely to be readmitted (RR 0.83; 95% CI 0.70 to 0.99) or die (RR 0.84; 95% CI 0.75 to 0.97) [81]. International experts agree, however, that such analyses need to take into

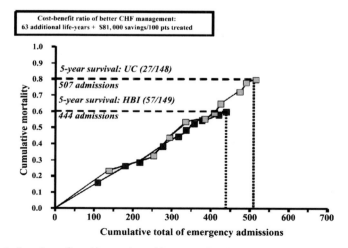

Figure 4.2 Cost-benefits of home-based intervention in CHF [80].

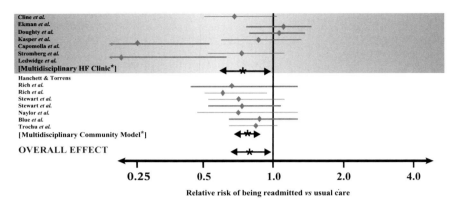

Figure 4.3 Overall benefits of multidisciplinary, CHF management [81].

account the specific intervention applied [82]. As such, using categories derived from an expert-consensus group, *a priori*, the various CHF programs of care were assigned to the following four categories of follow-up:
- Multidisciplinary, specialist CHF clinic (clinic-based intervention)
- Multidisciplinary, community-based management (home-based intervention)
- Remote management via telephone or interactive monitoring
- Education or self-care support [81,82].

The only models of care associated with a significant reduction in the risk of all-cause hospitalization were nurse-led, multidisciplinary clinic-, and home-based intervention (hazard plots shown in Figure 4.3) [81]. Home- and clinic-based interventions (RR 0.75; 95% CI 0.59 to 0.96) were also shown to reduce the risk of all-cause mortality: the former demonstrating the least amount of heterogeneity and providing the best outcomes overall. Remarkably, multidisciplinary management was shown to prevent a total of 160 events (comprising deaths and heart failure-related hospitalizations) compared to a 28 to 63 events/1000 patient years of treatment prevented by pharmacological agents [83]. Consequently, *all* four meta-analyses published in 2004 have called for appropriately powered, head-to-head studies of clinic and home-based multidisciplinary programs to decide which is most cost-effective in practice [81,84–86].

4.4 Reaching individuals living in rural and remote regions

As described above, meta-analyses have proven the effectiveness of multidisciplinary, CHF-MPs to improve the postdischarge management of CHF and substantially improve outcomes. However, with multifaceted approaches (more than one strategy) it has been difficult to identify if one or simply the combination of the treatments are effective [71,81]. What is significant is that within most populations there can be limited access to these programs for reasons such as economics and funding, or geography [87].

To meet the needs of CHF populations who are distal to CHF management programs, alternative models of care have been proposed and tested. These models have usually involved information communication technology (ICT) and have included telemonitoring (with transfer of data via digital cable relating to the patient's ECG, blood pressure, weight, oxygen saturation, respiratory rate, and medication adherence) or vigilance and support via a standard telephone, which may or may not include data transfer [88]. Both forms of monitoring can include the type of self-care and educational aspects described in greater detail in Chapter 6. For patients with CHF, self-management can play an important role in the maintenance or progression of disease irrespective of whether they live in rural and remote areas or not. In addition to treatment adherence, other behavioral parameters such as diet and exercise can impact on the burden of disease. Improved clinical outcomes for patients with CHF have previously been demonstrated following initiation of remote comprehensive patient care programs [88].

At the time of the first systematic review in this area by Louis and colleagues (published in 2003 [88]) it was suggested that telemonitoring for patients with CHF might have an important role as a part of a strategy for the delivery of effective health care and provide a means for keeping patients under close supervision, which could reduce the rate of admission and subsequent cost to the health care system. Unfortunately no adequately powered multicentered randomized controlled trials were available to evaluate the potential benefits. Subsequent to the Louis' review, McAlister and colleagues [81] reported that although standard telephone follow-up programs that advised deteriorating patients to see their regular physician do reduce CHF hospitalizations, they had no impact on mortality or all-cause hospitalization. These results were based on the 10 trials (1897 patients) that were available at the time [81]. In the time since the publication of these two important reviews several important reports have been published (DIAL [89], TENS-HMS [90], Benatar [91]), which may influence the results of earlier systematic reviews relating to the effectiveness of "remotely" managing CHF.

The Dial Trial found that telemonitoring was a low-cost intervention, which was effective in reducing the number and duration of heart failure admissions both in patients with mild (NYHA class I–II) and more severe (NYHA II–IV), and those with preserved ventricular function [89]. The TENS-HMS study in which 427 patients were randomized to usual care, nurse management (usual care plus monthly telephone calls), or telemonitoring (twice daily monitoring of vital signs), showed a substantial reduction in mortality compared to the usual care group [90], while Benatar has found that the adaptation of state of the art computer technology to closely monitor patients with HF via advanced practice nurse care is also likely to improve outcomes [91]. Table 4.1 outlines the most recent trials into this emerging area of CHF management.

Table 4.1 Recent trials of remote monitoring of patients with CHF.

Study (year)	N	Study population (location)	Mean age	Key components of intervention and outcomes	Duration of intervention
Pugh et al. (2001) [92]	58	Patients ≥65 years discharged from hospital with heart failure (US)	77	Nurse-led patient education, regular follow-up via telephone and clinic visits with nurse manager. Reduced HF-related hospitalization 0.98 (95% CI 0.49–1.98)	6 months
Jerant et al. (2001) [93]	37	Patients ≥40 years discharged from hospital with heart failure (US)	70	Nurse contact via telephone (mean 6 calls) or video-based home telecare (mean 9 calls), patient education, protocol-driven review of symptoms, medication compliance, and medication dosing, with communication to primary care physician if deterioration. Reduction in all cause mortality hospital admission and HF-related admission	2 months
de Lusignan et al. (2001) [94]	20	Adult patients with heart failure confirmed by cardiologist, identified from the database of an academic general practice (UK)	75	Telemonitoring of vital signs and clinical status daily, video consults with study nurse weekly × 3 months, biweekly × 3 months, then monthly. Reduction in all cause mortality hospital admission and HF-related admission	12 months
Riegel et al. (2002) [95]	358	Patients discharged from hospital with heart failure (US)	74	Nurse telephone contact (median 14 calls), patient education and counseling, case management guided by computer decision support, liaison with primary care physicians. Reduction in all cause mortality hospital admission and HF-related admission	6 months

Study	N	Population	Intervention / Outcomes	Duration
Laramee et al. (2003) [96]	287	Patients discharged from hospital with heart failure and having at least one risk factor for readmission (US)	Early discharge planning, patient education, regularly scheduled telephone contact (12 weeks, 9 calls), case manager sent reminders to primary care physician if not on target medications. Reduction in all cause mortality hospital admission and HF-related admission	3 months
Tsuyuki et al. (2004) [97]	276	Patients discharged from hospital with heart failure (Canada)	Early discharge planning with provision of adherence aids, patient education, regularly scheduled telephone contact (24 weeks, 7 calls) with recommendation to see primary care physician if not on target dose, ACE inhibitor, or deteriorated. Reduction in all cause mortality hospital admission and HF-related admission	6 months
Benatar 2003 [91]	216	Patients discharged from hospital with heart failure (USA)	Home nurse vs Telemonitoring. Reduced cost of care HF-related admission and LOS. Improved QOL.	3 months
DIAL Trial (2004) [89]	1518	Stable heart failure patients stabilized on medication (Argentina)	Intensive telephone intervention from trained nurse vs usual care. Calls made every 14 days for 4 calls then monthly. Low cost intervention reducing number and duration of HF-related admissions	12 months
TENS-HMS [90]	426	Patients recently admitted with CHF/ LVEF <40%	HTM (home telemonitoring) vs NTS (nurse telephone support) vs usual care 2:2:1. Substantial reduction in mortality in HTM and NTS compared to usual care.	3 months

4.5 Beyond heart failure: the potential to improve outcomes in other forms of chronic cardiac disease

In a recent meta-analysis of 102 studies evaluating the effectiveness of disease management programs, patient education and provider feedback were both associated with improvements in disease control [98]. Similarly, a review of home-based interventions targeting coronary heart disease also report improvements in disease control, a reduction in hospital admissions, and improvements in quality of life and functional status associated with these types of intervention strategies [99].

An increasing number of randomized studies of predominantly nurse-led programs of care have demonstrated that optimizing the postdischarge care of older patients with chronic disease can reduce the frequency of recurrent hospital use, improve quality of life, and even prolong survival in the process [100–102]. As exemplified by the data supporting CHF-MPs, the key components of the most successful programs are now well recognized:
- Multidisciplinary approach.
- Individualized care-based comprehensive needs assessment of clinical status, risk, and treatment.
- Patient education and counseling (often involving the family/carer).
- Intensive follow-up to detect and address clinical problems on a proactive basis.
- Strategies to both apply evidence-based pharmacological treatment and improve adherence.
- Lifestyle modification strategies (e.g. dietary and exercise).
- Patient-initiated access to appropriate advice and support.

In a recently reported pilot study, Inglis and colleagues [103] compared the pattern of recurrent hospitalization and mortality over five years in 152 patients with AF (53% male with a mean age of 73 ± 9 years) on the basis of the presence/absence of CHF and randomization to HBI or usual postdischarge care (UC). Consistent with previous data [77] and within the limits of Type II sample size error, those with concurrent CHF at baseline exposed to the CHF-specific form of HBI tended to have fewer readmissions, days of hospitalization, and fatal events relative to UC. In the absence of CHF, morbidity and mortality rates were significantly lower ($P < 0.001$) but still substantial during a five-year follow-up. In these patients, HBI was associated with prolonged event-free survival (34 vs 17 months: $P = 0.12$) and fewer fatal events (29% vs 53%: $P = 0.08$). HBI patients also had fewer readmissions (2.1 vs 2.6/patient) and days of hospitalization (16.3 vs 20.3/patient) compared to UC ($P = $ NS for both comparisons). On an adjusted basis, HBI was also associated with 30% fewer admissions for stroke, CHF, and AMI and 50% fewer admissions for respiratory failure, as outlined in Figure 4.4 [103].

Overall, these specific data, coupled with the extensive literature describing the benefits of individualized care in a heterogeneous range of chronic

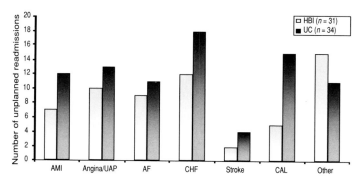

Figure 4.4 The effect of home-based intervention versus usual postdischarge care on unplanned readmissions in patients with chronic AF [116].

disease states (particularly those associated with the worst outcomes when managed within traditional health care programs) provide strong theoretical and practical reasons to more widely apply chronic cardiac care.

4.6 Summary

There is little doubt that predominantly nurse-led CHF-MPs can make a substantial impact on the lives of affected individuals and reduce costs in the process [104]. Supportive data from other chronic disease states (including chronic heart disease) suggest that if the following strategies used to develop and apply CHF-MPs were applied in more inclusive forms of chronic cardiac care, similar cost-benefits would be derived:

- Key involvement of specially trained cardiac nurses.
- Multidisciplinary approach.
- Specific targeting of a key condition(s) associated with suboptimal health outcomes related to poor application/uptake and high-risk for adverse events.
- Individualized approach to holistically manage health/disease with a strong focus on self-care.
- Well-developed strategic plans and management protocols.
- A commitment to continuous service improvement.
- Use of innovation to tackle specific issues/recalcitrant problems.

In the final section of this book (essentially putting all the evidence together), these key features are used to develop a "blueprint" for building an effective chronic cardiac care program or service. The next section of this book examines the types of specific issues and solutions relating to both the organization of the health care system and the individual patient that can be addressed and harnessed within the context of chronic cardiac care.

References

1 Gordon NF, Haskell W. Comprehensive cardiovascular disease risk reduction in a cardiac rehabilitation setting. A symposium: heart disease and heart failure. *Am J Cardiol* 1997; **80**(88):69H–73H.

2 World Health Organisation (WHO). Rehabilitation and comprehensive secondary prevention after acute myocardial infarction. Euro Report 1984. Copenhagen:1983.

3 Leon AS, Franklin BA, Costa F, et al. Cardiac rehabilitation and secondary prevention of coronary heart disease: an American Heart Association scientific statement from the Council on Clinical Cardiology in collaboration with the American Association of Cardiovascular and Pulmonary Rehabilitation. *Circulation* 2005; **111**(3):369–376.

4 Australian Cardiac Rehabilitation Association (ACRA), A practitioners guide to cardiac rehabilitation, ed. M.R.E. Services: Renard Marketing, Sydney, Australia, 1999.

5 O'Connor GT, Buring JE, Yusuf S, et al. An overview of randomized trials of rehabilitation with exercise after myocardial infarction. *Circulation* 1989; **80**(2):234–244.

6 Oldridge NB, Guyatt GH, Fischer ME, et al. Cardiac rehabilitation after myocardial infarction. Combined experience of randomized clinical trials. *JAMA* 1988; **260**(7):945–950.

7 Joliffe JA, Rees K, Taylor RS, et al. Exercise-based rehabilitation for coronary heart disease. Cochrane Review. In: The Cochrane Library, 2003; **1**:pp.1–41.

8 Giannuzzi P, Saner H, Bjornstad H, Giannuzzi P, et al. Secondary prevention through cardiac rehabilitation: position paper of the working group on cardiac rehabilitation and exercise physiology of the European Society of Cardiology. *Eur Heart J* 2003; **24**:1273–1278.

9 Taylor RS, Brown A, Ebrahim S, et al. Exercise-based rehabilitation for patients with coronary heart disease: systematic review and meta-analysis of randomized trials. *Am J Med* 2004; **116**:682–697.

10 Gordon NF, Salmon RD, Mitchell BS, et al. Innovative approaches to comprehensive cardiovascular disease risk reduction in clinical and community-based settings. *Curr Atheroscler Rep* 2001; **3**:498–506.

11 Daly J, Sindone AP, Thompson DR, et al. Barriers to participation in and adherence to cardiac rehabilitation programs: a critical literature review. *Prog Cardiovasc Nurs* 2002; **17**:8–17.

12 Andrew GM, Oldridge NB, Parker JO, et al. Reasons for dropout from exercise programs in post-coronary patients. *Med Sci Sports Exerc* 1981; **13**(3):164–168.

13 Ades PA, Waldmann ML, McCann WJ, et al. Predictors of cardiac rehabilitation participation in older coronary patients. *Arch Intern Med* 1992; **152**:1033–1035.

14 Gori P, Pivotti F, Mase N, et al. Compliance with cardiac rehabilitation in the elderly. *Eur Heart J* 1984; **5**(Suppl E):109–111.

15 Pell J, Pell A, Morrison C, et al. Retrospective study of influence of deprivation on uptake of cardiac rehabilitation. *BMJ* 1996; **313**(7052):267–268.

16 Petrie K J, Weinman J, Sharpe N, et al. Role of patients' view of their illness in predicting return to work and functioning after myocardial infarction: longitudinal study. *BMJ* 1996; **312**(7040):1191–1194.

17 Dracup K, Meleis A, Baker K, et al. Family-focused cardiac rehabilitation. A role supplementation program for cardiac patients and spouses. *Nurs Clin North Am* 1984; **19**(1):113–124.

18 Jackson L, Leclerc J, Erskine Y, et al. Getting the most out of cardiac rehabilitation: a review of referral and adherence patterns. *Heart* 2005; **91**:10–14.
19 Clark AM, Sharp C, MacIntyre PD. The role of age in moderating access to cardiac rehabilitation in Scotland. *Ageing Soc* 2002; **22**:501–515.
20 Clark AM, Barbour RS, White M, et al. Promoting participation in cardiac rehabilitation : patients' choices and experiences. *J Adv Nurs* 2004; **47**(1):5–14.
21 Oldridge NB. Compliance and exercise in primary and secondary prevention of coronary heart disease: a review. *Prev Med* 1982; **11**(1):56–70.
22 Fletcher GF, Balady G, Blair SN, et al. Statement on exercise: benefits and recommendations for physical activity programs for all Americans. A statement for health professionals by the Committee on Exercise and Cardiac Rehabilitation of the Council on Clinical Cardiology, American Heart Association. *Circulation* 1996; **94**(4): 857–862.
23 Frasure-Smith N, Prince R. The ischemic heart disease life stress monitoring program: impact on mortality. *Psychosom Med* 1985; **47**(Sept/Oct):431–445.
24 Wiles R. Empowering practice nurses in the follow-up of patients with established heart disease: lessons from patients' experiences. SHIP Collaborative Group. Southampton Heart Integrated Care Project. *J Adv Nurs* 1997; **26**(4): 729–735.
25 Wiles R. Patients' perceptions of their heart attack and recovery: the influence of epidemiological "evidence" and personal experience. *Soc Sci Med* 1998; **46**(11):1477–1486.
26 Wenger N, Froelicher E, Smith L, et al. Cardiac rehabilitation: clinical practice guideline No. 17, 1995. US Dept Health & Human Services, Public Health Service, Agency for Health Care Policy & Research, The National Heart, Lung, & Blood Institute: Rockville, MD.
27 Debusk RF, Haskell WL, Miller NH, et al. Multifit: A new system of coronary risk factor modification after acute myocardial infarction. In Proceedings of the 5th World Congress on Cardiac Rehabilitation (Bordeaux, France, 1992). Hampshire, UK: Intercept Ltd.
28 Bunker S, McBurney H, Cox H, et al. Identifying participation rates at outpatient cardiac rehabilitation programs in Victoria, Australia. *J Cardiopulm Rehabil* 1999; **19**:334–338.
29 Hawkes A. Predictors of health-related outcomes of heart disease after coronary bypass surgery or angioplasty in North Queensland, Australia. In: School of Public Health and Tropical Medicine. Townsville: James Cook University, 2000, p. 255.
30 Ades PA. Cardiac rehabilitation and secondary prevention of coronary heart disease. *N Engl J Med* 2001; **345**(12):892–902.
31 Pearson TA, Peters TD. The treatment gap in coronary artery disease and heart failure: community standards and the post-discharge patient. *Am J Cardiol* 1997; **80**(8B):45H–52H.
32 Brubaker P, Kaminsky L, Whaley M. *Coronary Artery Disease: essentials of prevention and rehabilitation programs.* Champaign: Human Kinetics, 2002.
33 Debusk RF, Miller NH, Superko R, et al. A case-management system for coronary risk factor modification after acute myocardial infarction. *Ann Intern Med* 1994; **120**(9):721–729.
34 Gordon NF, English CD, Contractor AS, et al. Effectiveness of three models for comprehensive cardiovascular disease risk reduction. *Am J Cardiol* 2002; **89**:1263–1268.

35 Southard BH, Southard DR, Nuckolls J. Clinical trial of an internet-based case management system for secondary prevention of heart disease. *J Cardiopulm Rehabil* 2003; **23**:341–348.

36 Debusk RF, Haskell WL, Miller NH, et al. Medically directed at-home rehabilitation soon after clinically uncomplicated myocardiac infarction: a new model for patient care. *Am J Cardiol* 1985; **55**:251–257.

37 Beckie T. A supportive-educative telephone program: impact on knowledge and anxiety after coronary artery bypass graft surgery. *Heart & Lung* 1989; **18**:46–55.

38 Lewin B, Roberston I, Cay E, et al. Effects of self-help post-myocardial-infarction rehabilitation on psychological adjustment and use of health services. *Lancet* 1992; **339**:1036–1040.

39 Debusk RF, Haskell WL, Miller NH, et al. Multifit: a new system of coronary risk factor modification after acute myocardial infarction. In: *Proceedings of the 5th World Congress on Cardiac Rehabilitation.* Hampshire, UK: Intercept Ltd.

40 Haskell WL, Alderman EL, Fair J, et al. Effects of intensive multiple risk factor reduction on coronary atherosclerosis and clinical cardiac events in men and women with coronary artery disease. The Stanford Coronary Risk Intervention Project. *Circulation* 1994; **39**(3):975–990.

41 Johnston M, Foulkes J, Johnston DW, et al. Impact on patients and partners of inpatient and extended cardiac counselling and rehabilitation: a controlled trial. *Psychosom Med* 1999; **61**:225–233.

42 Ades PA, Pashkow FJ, Fletcher G, et al. A controlled trial of cardiac rehabilitation in the home setting using electrocardiographic and voice transtelephonic monitoring. *Am Heart J* 2000; **139**:543–548.

43 Higgins HC, Hayes RL, McKenna KT. Rehabilitation outcomes following percutaneous coronary interventions (PCI). *Patient Educ Couns* 2001; **43**:219–230.

44 Jolly K, Lip GYH, Sandercock J, et al. Home-based versus hospital-based cardiac rehabilitation after myocardial infarction or revascularisation: design and rationale of the Birmingham rehabilitation uptake maximisation study (BRUM): a randomised controlled trial. *BMC Cardiovasc Disord* 2003; **3**:1–11.

45 Vale MJ, Jelinek MV, Grigg LE, et al. Coaching patients on achieving cardiovascular health (COACH): a multicentre randomised trial in patients with coronary heart disease. *Arch Intern Med* 2003; **163**:2775–2783.

46 Brubaker PH, Rejeski WJ, Smith MJ, et al. A home-based maintenance exercise program after center-based cardiac rehabilitation: effects on blood lipids, body composition, and functional capacity. *J Cardiopulm Rehabil* 2000; **20**:(1)50–56.

47 Hamm LF, Kavanagh T, Campbell RB, et al. Timeline for peak improvements during 52 weeks of outpatient cardiac rehabilitation. *J Cardiopulm Rehabil* 2004; **24**:374–382.

48 Fonarow G, Gawlinski A, Moughrabi S, et al. Improved treatment of coronary heart disease by implementation of a cardiac hospitalisation atherosclerosis management program (CHAMP). *Am J Cardiol* 2001; **87**:819–822.

49 DeBusk RF, West JA, Miller NH, et al. Chronic disease management: treating the patient with disease(s) vs treating disease(s) in the patient. *Arch Intern Med* 1999; **159**(22):2739–2742.

50 Linden B. Evaluation of a home-based rehabilitation programme for patients recovering from acute myocardial infarction. *Intensive Crit Care Nurs* 1995; **11**:10–19.

51 O'Rourke A, Hampson S. Psychosocial outcomes after an MI: an evaluation of two approaches to rehabilitation. *Psychology, Health and Medicine* 1999; **4**:393–402.

52 Lacey EA, Musgrave RJ, Freeman JV, et al. Psychological morbidity after myocardial infarction in an area of deprivation in the UK: evaluation of a self-help package. *Eur J Cardiovasc Nurs* 2004; **3**(3):219–224.

53 Dalal HM, Evans PH. Achieving national service framework standards for cardiac rehabilitation and secondary prevention. *BMJ* 2003; **326**:481–484.

54 Shaw DK, Heggestad-Hereford JR, Southard DR, et al. American Association of Cardiovascular and Pulmonary Rehabilitation Telemedicine Position Statement. *J Cardiopulm Rehabil* 2001; **21**:261–262.

55 American Nurses Association. *Handbook of Nursing Case Management.* Gaithersburg, MD: Aspen Publishers, 1996.

56 Unger BT, Warren DA. Case management in cardiac rehabilitation. In: Wenger NK, et al., eds. *Cardiac Rehabilitation: a guide to practice in the 21st century.* New York: Marcel Dekker,1999, pp. 327–341.

57 Wilson BT, Foresman J. You can help your patients cope: why coaching and not training. In American association of cardiovascular and pulmonary rehabilitation. Long Beach, California, 2004.

58 Franklin BA, Bonzheim K, Gordon S, et al. Safety of medically supervised cardiac rehabilitation exercise therapy: a 16-year follow-up. *Chest* 1998; **114**:902–906.

59 Lear SA, Ignaszewski A. Cardiac rehabilitation: a comprehensive review. *Curr Control Trials Cardiovasc Med* 2001; **2**(5):221–232.

60 Weingarten SR, Henning JM, Badamgarav E, et al. Interventions used in disease management programmes for patients with chronic illness–which ones work? Meta-analysis of published reports. *BMJ* 2002; **325**(7370):925.

61 Theis SL, Johnson JH. Strategies for teaching patients: a meta-analysis. *Clin Nurse Spec* 1995; **9**(2):100–105, 120.

62 O'Connor AM, Stacey D, Entwistle V, et al. Decision aids for people facing health treatment or screening decisions (Cochrane Review). In: *The Cochrane Library,* Issue 1. Chichester, UK: Wiley & Sons, 2004.

63 National Health Service. Informing, communication and sharing decisions with people who have cancer. *Eff Health Care* 2000; **6**(6):1–8.

64 Coulter, A. Evidence-based patient information. is important, so there needs to be a national strategy to ensure it. *BMJ* 1998; **317**(7153):225–226.

65 Lear S, Ignaszewski A, Linden W, et al. The extensive lifestyle management intervention (ELMI) following cardiac rehabilitation trial. *Eur Heart J* 2003; **24**:1920–1927.

66 Moore SM, Ruland CM, Pashkow FJ, et al. Women's patterns of exercise following cardiac rehabilitation. *Nurs Res* 1998; **47**:318–324.

67 Willich SN, Muller-Nordhorn J, Kulig M, et al. Cardiac risk factors, medication, and recurrent clinical events after acute coronary disease; a prospective cohort study. *Eur Heart J* 2001; **22**:307–313.

68 Labrador MP, Merz CNB, Pass R. A randomized trial of risk factor case management in coronary artery disease patients following cardiac rehabilitation (Abstr). *Circulation* 1998; **98**:1811

69 Tunstall-Pedoe H, Kuulasmaa K, Mahonen M, et al. Contribution of trends in survival and coronary-event rates to changes in coronary heart disease mortality: 10-year results from 37 WHO MONICA Project populations. *Lancet* 1999; **353**:1547–1557.

70 Yusuf S, Sleight P, Pogue J, et al. Effects of an angiotensin-converting enzyme inhibitor, ramipril, on cardiovascular events in high-risk patients. The heart

outcomes prevention evaluation study investigators. *N Engl J Med* 2001; **342**:145–153.

71 Moser K, Mann DL. Improving outcomes in heart failure: it's not unusual beyond usual care. *Circulation* 2002; **105**:2810–2812.

72 Gattis WA, Hasselblad V, Whellan DJ, et al. Reduction in heart failure events by the addition of a clinical pharmacist to the heart failure management team: results of the Pharmacist in Heart Failure Assessment Recommendation and Monitoring (PHARM) Study. *Arch Intern Med* 1999; **159**:1939–1945.

73 Rich MW, Beckham V, Wittenberg C, et al. A multidisciplinary intervention to prevent the readmission of elderly patients with congestive heart failure. *New Engl J Med* 1995; **333**:1190–1195.

74 Stewart S, Pearson S, Luke CG, et al. Effects of a home based intervention on unplanned readmissions and out-of-hospital deaths. *J Am Geriatr Soc* 1998; **46**:174–180.

75 Stewart S, Pearson S, Horowitz JD. Effects of a home-based intervention among patients with chronic congestive heart failure. *Arch Intern Med* 1998; **158**:1067–1072.

76 Stewart S, Vandenbroek A, Pearson S, et al. Prolonged beneficial effects of a home-based intervention on unplanned readmissions and mortality among congestive heart failure patients. *Arch Intern Med* 1999; **159**:257–261.

77 Stewart S, Marley JE, Horowitz JD. Effects of a multidisciplinary, home-based intervention on unplanned readmissions and survival among patients with chronic congestive heart failure: a randomized controlled study. *Lancet* 1999; **354**:1077–1083.

78 Swedberg K, Kjekshus J, Snapinn S, for the CONSENSUS investigators. Long-term survival in severe heart failure in patients with enalapril. *Eur Heart J* 1999; **20**:136–139.

79 Stewart S, Horowitz JD. Home-based intervention in congestive heart failure: long-term implications on readmission and survival. *Circulation* 2002; **105**:2861–2866.

80 Inglis S, Horowitz JD, Stewart S. Long-term cost-effectiveness of a nurse-led, home-based intervention in chronic heart failure. *Heart Lung & Circulation* 2004; **13**:S2–S9.

81 McAlister FA, Stewart S, Ferrua J, et al. Multidisciplinary strategies for the management of heart failure patients a high-risk admission: a systematic review of randomised trials. *J Am Coll Cardiol* 2004; **44**:810–819.

82 Riegel B, Naylor M, Stewart S, et al. Interventions to prevent readmission for congestive heart failure (Scientific Letter). *JAMA* 2004;**16**:291.

83 Flather MD, Yusuf S, Kober L, et al. Long-term ACE inhibitor therapy in patients with heart failure or left ventricular dysfunction: a systematic overview of data from individuals patients. *Lancet* 2000; **355**:1575–1581.

84 Phillips CO, Wright SM, Kern DE, et al. Comprehensive discharge planning with post discharge support for older patients with congestive heart failure: a meta-analysis. *JAMA* 2004; **291**(11):1358–1367.

85 Gonseth J, Guallar-Castillon P, Banegas JR, et al. The effectiveness of disease management programmes in reducing hospital re-admission in older patients with heart failure: systematic review and meta-analysis of published reports. *Eur Heart J* 2004; **25**(18):1570–1595.

86 Gwadry-Sridhar FH, Flintoft V, Lee DS, et al. A systematic review and meta-analysis of studies comparing readmission rates and mortality rates *Arch Intern Med* 2004; **64**:2315–2320.

87 Clark RA, Driscoll A, Nottage J, et al. Overcoming the tyranny of distance: a mis-match of supply and demand for specialist chronic heart failure management in Australia2005 Submitted to *Eur J Heart Failure* 2005.

88 Louis AA, Turner T, Gretton M, et al. A systematic review of telemonitoring for the management of heart failure. *Eur J Heart Fail* 2003; **5**:585–590.

89 Collette AP, Nikitin N, Clark AL, et al. Clinical trials update from the American Heart Association meeting: PROSPER, DIAL, home telemonitoring trials, immune modulation therapy, COMPANION and anaemia in heart failure. *Eur J Heart Fail* 2003; **5**:95–99.

90 Cleland JGF, Louis AA, Rigby AS,et al. The Trans-European Network-Home-Care Management System (TENS-HMS) Study. Noninvasive home telemonitoring for patients with heart failure at high risk of recurrent admission and death. *JACC* 2005; **45**(10):1654–1664.

91 Benetar D, Bondmass M, Ghitelman J, et al. Outcomes of chronic heart failure. *Arch Intern Med* 2003; **163**:347–352.

92 Pugh LC, Havens DS, Xie S, et al. Case management for elderly persons with heart failure: the quality of life and cost outcomes. *MedSurg Nursing* 2001;10:71-78.

93 Jerant AF, Azari R, Nesbitt T. Reducing the cost of frequent hospital admissions for congestive heart failure. *Med Care* 2001; **39**:1234–1245.

94 de Lusignan S, Wells S, Johnson P, et al. Compliance and effectiveness of 1 year's home telemonitoring. The report of a pilot study of patients with chronic heart failure. *Eur J Heart Fail* 2001; **3**:723–730.

95 Reigel B, Carlson B, Kopp Z, et al. Efficacy of a standardised nurse case management telephone intervention on resource use in patients with chronic heart failure. *Arch Intern Med* 2002; **162**:705–712.

96 Laramee A, Levinsky SK, Sargent J, et al. Case management in a heterogenous congestive heart failure population: a randomized controlled trial. *Arch Intern Med* 2003; **163**:809–817.

97 Tsuyuki RT, McKelvie RS, Arnold JM, et al. Acute precipitants of congestive heart failure exacerbations. *Arch Intern Med* 2001; **161**:2337–2342.

98 Weingarten SR, Henning JM, Badamgarav E, et al. Interventions used in disease management programmes for patients with chronic illness–which ones work? Meta-analysis of published reports. *BMJ* 2002; **325**:925.

99 Elkan R, Kendrick D, Dewey M, et al. Effectiveness of home-based support for older people: systematic review and meta-analysis. *BMJ* 2001; **323**:719–725.

100 Col N, Fanale JE, Kronholm P. The role of medication noncompliance and adverse drug reactions in hospitalizations of the elderly. *Arch Intern Med* 1990; **150**:841–845.

101 McAlister FA, Lawson FM, Teo KK, et al. Randomized trials of secondary preven-tion programmes in coronary heart disease: systematic review. *BMJ* 2001; **323**:957–962.

102 Ofman JJ, Badamgarav E, Henning JM, et al. Does disease management inprove clinical and economic outcomes in patients with chronic disease? A systematic review. *Am J Med* 2004; **117**:182–192.

103 Inglis SC, Dawson AP, Wilkinson D, et al. A new solution to an old problem? Effects of a nurse-led, home-based intervention in chronic atrial fibrillation. *Eur Heart J* 2003; **24**:484.

104 Weintraub WS, Cole J, Tooley JF. Cost and cost-effectiveness studies in heart failure research. *Am Heart J* 2002; **143**:565–576.

Section 3
Managing Care: From the Organization to the Individual

CHAPTER 5

Organizational aspects of chronic cardiac care

5.1 Introduction

The typically poor health outcomes associated with chronic cardiac disease described in Chapter 1 should come as no surprise given the progressive nature of heart disease with age, and the inherently complex interaction between the individual, their treatment, and the many components of the health care system within which they are managed. Anything that interrupts or hinders what should be a harmonious and productive interaction between the patient and the health care system has the potential to lead to less than optimal outcomes at the individual level and, through a process equivalent to a "death by a thousand cuts," a dysfunctional health care system. Clearly, the models of secondary prevention designed to limit the progression of underlying heart disease described in Chapter 3, and the models of chronic disease management (in particular CHF) described in Chapter 4, when combined, offer a practical and cost-effective means to improve outcomes at the individual and population level. However, the inherent difficulties in translating successful research programs or, indeed, applying established services that have been successfully applied within a "foreign" health care system (e.g. a managed care environment with capped levels of service provision) cannot be overstated. The ultimate aim, of course, is to ensure that the quality of service provided to patients, whatever its format, is consistently maintained at the highest possible standard over a prolonged period, irrespective of its location and the individuals involved. This requires the efforts of a dedicated team prepared to invest an enormous amount of time and energy to establish the highest possible standards of care. It also requires a good understanding of the organizational framework (i.e. the key components that cannot be neglected) that will form the basis of a cost-effective service. It is within this context that this chapter examines and outlines the key components of services to improve management of chronic cardiac conditions.

5.2 Essential ingredients for establishing a service

Prior to establishing a formal service and considering any of the finer details of patient management, it is essential that a core, dedicated team reviews the available evidence, the needs of the local patient population, and the overall health care environment, to undertake the critical steps outlined below. This is obviously best undertaken under the auspices of a powerful advocacy (e.g. the National Institute of Clinical Studies in Australia), professional (European Society of Cardiology), or charitable organization (American Heart Association), dedicated to translating good research into practice. The essential ingredients for establishing a service include the following steps.

Formulate an overall strategy to fund and organize the service

Devise a strategy to present to the local, regional, or national Health Department or Authority with the power to fund and implement the proposed initiative: this is easier to achieve if there is a good evidence base (see Chapters 3 and 4). The proposed initiative should underpin local implementation of any national (e.g. the National Service Framework in the United Kingdom) or professional (the American Heart Association's "Get with the Guidelines") guidelines and reinforce national initiatives to combat an epidemic of heart disease in ageing Western populations. As part of this process, it is advisable to undertake the following:

- Interest a few enthusiasts and influential leaders.
- Identify stakeholders and form a steering group with representation from all stakeholder groups, health care professionals, and managers from hospitals and the community (ensure all stakeholders are involved).
- Undertake (if possible) a pilot program to show the service can work and provide tangible cost-benefits: this is often essential to secure sufficient resources.
- Plan for a sustainable service with recurrent funding from the beginning.
- Doubly ensure that the model of care suits the local health care environment and patient population.

Define the service

Based on the above, it is essential to define the key features of the service in a clear and precise manner. As such, it is important to:

- Identify the most important health priorities and agree on the primary (and secondary) purpose of the service in terms of short- and long-term health outcomes.
- Develop precise and realistic aims and objectives.
- Draw up clear protocols and guidelines that have been agreed by all the key stakeholders and that reflect local and national guidelines.
- Define referral criteria – which patients, how will they be referred?
- Develop mechanisms to identify eligible patients and how they will be referred to the service.
- Ensure support from key players (e.g. GP/primary care physician and hospital physician).
- Calculate likely patient caseloads during the critical process of establishing the service, at "steady state" (i.e. when the balance between recruitment/

management of active patients versus loss of patients via fatal events or discharge has stabilized), and in the longer-term.
- Identify the number and type of specialist nurses required to manage the projected number of patients.
- Identify the infrastructure, support services, and personnel that will need to be dedicated to the service in addition to its likely impact on preexisting health care and social support services.

Identify practical issues of implementation

During the process of developing a new service it is always tempting to become carried away with grandiose plans to cover every health contingency and to overestimate its overall impact. Adopting a pragmatic approach is therefore essential, particularly when funding and resources are likely to be limited. This would include:
- Applying an incremental approach to ensure that teething problems are immediately identified and addressed as they occur.
- Establish formal links with other relevant health care services.
- Clarify the role of other potentially affected health care professionals to avoid inappropriate referrals.
- Ensure cooperation from all relevant health care professionals and administrators (not just the "enthusiasts"!).
- Clearly identify the limitations of the local health care system to prevent overloading health care services with additional and unrealistic demands.
- Conversely, identify preexisting initiatives (e.g. in Australia there is now Federal funding of multidisciplinary care plans, management conferences, and various forms of health care contracts arising from such activities).
- Develop various forms (i.e. written literature to interactive forms based on multimedia formats) of patient information.
- Plan for regular evaluation and auditing of service provision and outcomes.
- Plan for the regular review of service protocols and guidelines to keep abreast of new research and guidelines.
- Develop specific tools to monitor both patient and carer satisfaction levels.
- Establish realistic plans for service expansion and development based on a range of scenarios (e.g. increasing versus diminishing need for active intervention).

Establish ideal budget and resources

Clearly nothing is likely to happen without realistic budgets and financial projections showing the positive impact of the service in the short, medium, and longer-term. Sadly, it is no longer possible to apply successful health care strategies without considering the costs! Fortunately, as shown in Chapter 1, there is an urgent need to tackle the enormous cost of dealing with the unacceptably high levels of morbidity associated with chronic cardiac disease. Specialist nurse-led programs of care are likely to be extremely cost-effective whenever the focus of care is shifted from acute hospital care and expensive

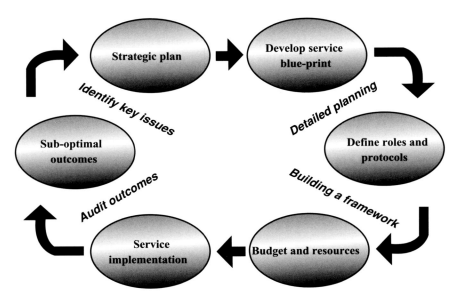

Figure 5.1 Improving health outcomes in chronic cardiac disease: the continuous cycle of strategic planning and improvement.

invasive procedures in favor of community-focussed health care. Key components of cost will include:
- Cost for salary of specialist nurses (built in cover for sickness, annual leave, study leave, etc.)
- Office and/or clinic space and equipment.
- Transport (e.g. supplying a car with ongoing travel costs).
- Communication (e.g. phone, mobile phone, fax, paperwork, computing).
- Equipment (e.g. weighing scales, venepuncture equipment, computer equipment).
- Additional investigations (e.g. laboratory costs).
- Referral costs to other professionals (e.g. dietician, pharmacist, social worker, audit personnel, information technology support).
- Patient information books.
- Training costs (e.g. an induction program, ongoing training and development).

Figure 5.1 demonstrates that the process of developing a cost-effective health care program/service requires a continuous cycle of strategic planning and improvement based on the key ingredients listed above.

5.3 Summary

Effective chronic cardiac care is not applied in a vacuum. In many cases, efforts to apply the principles of good management and effective therapy outlined in this book will be attempted within an already dysfunctional health care system or specific organization. In order to succeed in the longer-term, the therapeutic benefits of applying an individual approach to managing chronic cardiac care has to be nested within a supportive framework (whether it be within a larger organization or as a "stand-alone" service) that clearly articulates who will be managed, how they will be managed, how the specialist cardiac nurses, patients, and their carers will articulate with other parts of the health care system, and what specific outcomes are expected from the health care program/service when appropriately audited and assessed. As summarized in this chapter, the answers to these questions are best derived from a critical analysis of the strength and weaknesses of the local health care system and thorough planning. It is within this context that the next chapter addresses the other side of the health care equation – what motivates and drives individual patients to react in the way they do to their own health and the health care delivered to them.

CHAPTER 6
Individual aspects of chronic cardiac care

6.1 Introduction

In the absence of the critical analysis and strategic planning outlined in Chapter 5, there is a tendency for health care systems, regional services, and individual programs alike to adopt the "patient factory" approach and manage patients according to their nominal diagnosis rather than on an individual basis. However, no one patient is the same as the next in terms of their life-experiences, personality, and beliefs. Moreover, their personal experience and interpretation of the "same" diagnosis and interaction with the health care system will vary markedly. Hence numerous studies (as outlined in Section 2) have highlighted that the key to improving clinical outcomes, reducing hospital admissions, and improving the quality of life of individual patients with chronic cardiac disease is holistically based, multidisciplinary programs of care that often involve interventions that focus on tailoring health care to the individual rather than constraining such care to suit impositions set by the health care system (e.g. caring for patients outside of the traditional hospital setting).

Management of the chronic cardiac conditions, chronic angina pectoris, CHF, and AF is a complex, tiring, and time-consuming process that continues for the patient day in and day out. Not only is there a great deal of variation in the clinical condition of each patient, but there is also often a complex array of individual responses to being confronted with a bewildering list of treatments and strategies to manage their condition. This process is not made any easier by the fact that many patients are elderly (with potential cognitive impairment), are suffering from debilitating symptoms, and have to deal with a life-time of habits that conspire against adopting new ways to manage their health and illness. It is within this context that the emergence of an epidemic of chronic cardiac disease has necessitated the development of intensive and individualized approaches to enable those afflicted to manage medications, lifestyle, and dietary strategies, whilst simultaneously attempting to maintain or improve quality of life.

These individualized programs of care are largely based on the education of the patient about their illness, medications, diet, and how to recognize and manage exacerbations of their condition – that is, developing programs of *self-management*. In defining self-management Bodenheimer and colleagues

(2002) [1] state that "self-management education compliments traditional patient education in supporting patients to live the best quality of life with their chronic condition" [1]. Lorig 1996 [2] differentiates between programs of self-care, self-help, and self-management by asserting that true self-management education must employ five key criteria:

1 Content that is focussed on the individual's perceived needs.
2 Practice and feedback in new skills such as decision making and problem solving.
3 Awareness of emotional and role management in addition to medical management.
4 Employing techniques to improve an individual's confidence in their own ability to manage their conditions.
5 Placing an emphasis on the individual's active role in the doctor/patient relationship [2].

The effects of these types of programs are believed to be mediated via the impact on the individual's self-efficacy, or perceived control over their disease process [2,3]. In order to effectively provide education to the individual about their condition and, in order for them to self-manage that condition, an understanding of the key concepts of health education is valuable for the health professional undertaking this role. The key strategies are outlined in this chapter.

This chapter, therefore, focusses on the individual aspects of care for chronic cardiac conditions and considers fundamental components such as holistic approaches to therapy, adherence to therapy, and finally discusses five theories of health psychology that may assist the health care professional to develop and implement education to improve care in individuals. Whilst there are examples of how these theories relate to chronic cardiac conditions, the actual education and best practice guidelines contained in such a self-management program is outlined in previous sections of this book, and simply must be adapted to suit the situation.

6.2 Holistic approach and impact of the illness on the person

Chronic cardiac disease imposes not only a physical burden on the patient, but also a significant psychological burden, a factor which may often be overlooked due to the significance and degree of the patient's physical symptoms of the illness. Depression and anxiety have been associated with all three common forms of chronic cardiac disease, which forms the major focus of this book [4–9], often leaving the patient physically exhausted and unmotivated due to physical symptoms and psychological effects (such as disturbed sleep). This physical and psychological burden often imparts its load not only on the patient, but also on significant others such as carers [10], family, and friends.

Whilst there is a significant psychological burden on all patients with chronic disease, it has been reported that between the genders, differences may exist in the individual's approach to the limitations and burden of the condition [11], with women demonstrating better psychosocial adjustment to illness than men [12]. It may be necessary, therefore, to tailor patient teaching and counseling to address gender specific issues [12]. As an example of the impact of chronic cardiac disease on an individual's qualify of life, Evangelista and colleagues [12] reported four major themes (outlined below in no particular order) in analyzing patients with CHF responses to the following question: "how has your condition affected your life?"

- Physical impairment (decreased functional ability and vitality, symptom distress, side effects of treatment).
- Emotional burden (fear/uncertainty, hopelessness, depression, anger, anxiety).
- Role limitations (unable to work, unable to meet family roles, poor self concept, social limitations).
- Loss (loss of independence, health and control, and financial losses).

To enable the success of an appropriate and effective individual intervention to promote self-care in patients with a chronic cardiac condition the health care professional must consider the whole person and address not only their physical, but also their psychological symptoms and needs. Once such an approach is mastered, improvements in the individual's health outcomes, most probably brought about by better adherence to treatment programs, may be evident.

6.3 Adherence to programs

Treatment adherence is akin to compliance but does not suggest the paternalistic interpretations of compliance. Thus, for this reason adherence, rather than compliance to treatment, is discussed. To outline this issue definitions for both terms are provided.

Compliance. Considered to be a measurement of the concordance between the prescribed treatment and the subsequent behavior of the individual [13]. The Hasting Report on Ethical Challenges in Chronic Illness (1988) outlines that a contractual agreement exists between the provider (health care professional) and the patient [14].

Adherence. The World Health Organisation (2003) [15] defines adherence as: "...the extent to which a person's behavior-taking medication, following a diet, and/or executing lifestyle changes corresponds with agreed recommendations from a provider" [15].

Concordance. Another frequently used term in this context; concordance has been discussed in some literature and may be described as a therapeutic alliance between the patient and the health care professional [16].

As outlined by these definitions of compliance, adherence, and concordance to the management of chronic cardiac disease relates not only to pharmacological treatment, but also dietary modifications, exercise, rehabilitation programs, and lifestyle adaptations. For example, in the following specific conditions:

- Chronic angina pectoris – maintaining and reducing a lower risk factor profile for further cardiac events.
- CHF – adherence to behaviors such as reduced sodium intake, daily weighing, monitoring of fluid balance, and smoking cessation.
- AF – managing anticoagulation, reducing fatigue, and monitoring symptoms, along with general issues for all conditions such as exercise, alcohol reduction, and weight management.

Positive evidence for the benefit of self-management in these conditions is present in the literature, highlighted by just one example of self-management in AF. Self-management of anticoagulation has been demonstrated to improve outcomes by maintaining such therapy within therapeutic boundaries and reducing the incidence of bleeding complications and thromboembolic events [17–20]. In this context, the use of portable prothrombin time monitors has increased patient responsibility for managing anticoagulation [21]. Furthermore, a study specifically investigating prothrombin time testing at home by elderly patients with chronic AF reported that the more frequent testing as done by those self-managing their oral anticoagulation provided better results [21] and alleviated the need to attend clinics, improved compliance (sic), and allowed proper dosage adjustment of oral anticoagulants [21]. This issue of adherence to medical treatments in chronic conditions is not easily solved, as many factors contribute to poor adherence, not all necessarily related to the individual or to medication mismanagement.

Whilst collection methods vary between studies, adherence rates have been reported as poor in those not included in specific management programs or clinics. For example, in a general CHF patient population, it was found that only 10% were found to be fully compliant with prescribed treatment [22]. Similarly, Cline and colleagues found the following, in a similar patient cohort of elderly CHF patients that:

- 55% correctly named what medication had been prescribed
- 50% were unable to state the prescribed doses
- 64% could not account for what medication was to be taken
- overall, 73% were compliant (sic) with their prescribed medication regimen [23].

There are many contributing factors when considering adherence to medication regimes, and a key factor can be the number of dosing periods during a day, which has been demonstrated to correlate to decreased adherence to the regime [24]. Whilst adherence is an issue for any chronic disease management, disease-specific programs of care have been shown to improve adherence to both pharmacologic and other treatment and lifestyle adaptations; for example, Ni and colleagues (1999) [25] reported medication adherence levels of 71–74% for those enrolled in specific CHF clinics.

As has been continually indicated throughout this book many interacting factors impact on adherence to treatment programs. This fact cannot be

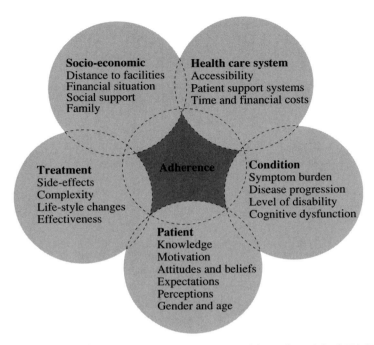

Figure 6.1 The five dimensions of adherence. (Adapted from the original [13,15].)

overstated. The WHO report on adherence outlines five dimensions that interact to affect the compliance of each individual to their program as outlined in Figure 6.1 [15]. The five dimensions and some of the possible contributing factors are outlined below [13,15].

In order to improve adherence to treatment regimes, interventions must target these barriers outlined and any intervention must not solely rely on patient orientated factors to adherence, but consider all five dimensions affecting it [15]. In consideration of this chapter and its focus on individual aspects of managing chronic cardiac conditions, it is highlighted that the "patient" dimension of the WHO model is strongly linked to components of various health psychology theories, which is explored later in this chapter.

Given the vast differences in patients' understanding of their illness and management, it is important to assess the patient's adherence, knowledge, and understanding of their overall management program (pharmacological, dietary, lifestyle, etc.). It is also important to consider the often critical role of carers who frequently manage the patient's medications, diet, and appointments. Thus, any intervention or education must include not only the patient but also the person who assumes the day-to-day management of the therapeutic regimen. All the while, such interventions should encompass and promote self-care and management within the constraints of the individual's cognitive ability. The interrelated concepts of adherence and knowledge may be considered diagrammatically as represented by Figure 6.2 [26]. This is a

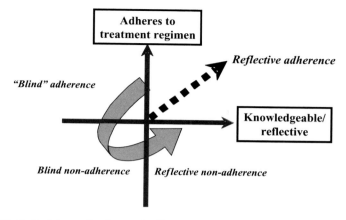

Figure 6.2 Optimizing reflection and adherence. (Adapted from the original [27].)

conceptualization of treatment adherence and knowledge that was developed from patterns identified in a large cohort of chronically ill patients [26].

Figure 6.2 outlines the need to consider the two components of treatment knowledge and awareness and adherence separately. This excerpt from a previous text specifically focusses on the role, critical reflection, and adherence in improving outcomes in those with CHF, but has the same relevance to those with other forms of chronic cardiac disease:

> For example, to the knowledgeable it would appear inadvisable to strictly adhere to prescribed high dose ACE inhibition when feeling increasingly dizzy, fatigued and, despite drinking reasonable amounts of water, finding no desire to void, yet such "blind adherence" is common and much less desirable than "reflective nonadherence" based on a sound knowledge of the risk-benefits of a prescribed regimen a reasoned decision not to follow medical/nursing advice. Ideally, most patients could be "trained" and motivated to practice "reflective adherence" to their treatment. However, in practical terms we often have to make do with applying strategies that provide a "safety net" to protect them against adverse effects and maximise potential benefits, knowing that rates of adherence and benefit are inversely related to the number of doses prescribed: i.e. the greater the potential for something to go wrong, the more likely it will go wrong! [26]

6.4 Education to promote self-management – health psychology models

Within the context of providing necessary and effective education to individuals to support and encourage self-management and to improve adherence to treatment programs, several health promotion, and nursing theories have identified a number of key determinates of health and illness at the individual level. Any one of these theories may be applied to improve the chronic cardiac conditions outlined in this book: consistent with the overall philosophy underlying this book, the authors propose an eclectic adoption of the most pragmatic and effective principals underlying these theories and models be applied at the individual level. Four main health promotion theories (Health Belief Model, Social-Cognitive/Social Learning Theory, Theory of Reasoned Action, and Transtheoretical/Stages of Change Model) are outlined along with a nursing-specific theory (Orem's General Theory of Nursing), and their application to the management of both the symptoms of the condition and reducing the risk of further events, is discussed.

Health belief model

The Health Belief Model, developed by Becker in 1974 [28] proposes that an individual's belief about a particular behavior will predict their actual behavior [29]. The fundamental component of this theory is the concept that "...the likelihood of an individual taking action related to a given health problem is based on the interaction between four different types of belief" [30]. These four belief types, (i) perceived susceptibility, (ii) perceived seriousness, (iii) perceived benefits, and (iv) perceived barriers, are based on the individual's perception of the relevance of the threat or outcome to themselves and are related to their own self-efficacy or their belief in their own self to undertake a change to their health behavior [30]. The four perceived belief types and their application to chronic atrial fibrillation are outlined in Figure 6.3 [30].

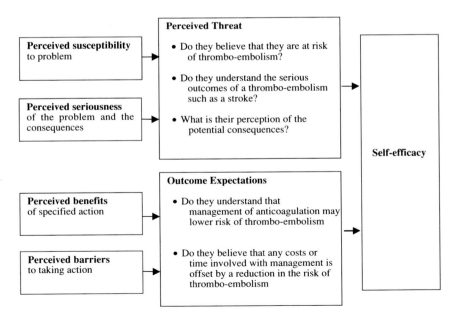

Figure 6.3 The health belief model in action: chronic atrial fibrillation. (Adapted from the original [30].)

A review of this model demonstrates the explicit contribution of other factors, besides those relating to the psychosocial context of the individual (most notably attitudes and beliefs) in influencing health-related behaviors and subsequent outcomes [31]. Other factors to consider include access to adequate resources, lifestyle barriers, and socioeconomic deprivation.

Health belief model and research on adherence

This model has been applied to evaluate CHF patients' beliefs about adherence [29] and has been used by other researchers to investigate adherence-related health problems in health promotion and management of noncardiac conditions [32,33]. Bennett and colleagues [29] tested the reliability and validity of two scales adapted from the health belief model to investigate CHF patient's beliefs about medication and dietary adherence, concluding that the "Health Belief Model is a useful framework for evaluating beliefs about compliance among patients with heart failure" [29]. Dunbar and colleagues [34] suggest that using an example of heart failure management the Health Belief Model could be used to:

> ...direct the nurse to assess the patient's view of the positive benefits he or she could achieve from such habits as eating a low sodium diet, restricting fluids, taking medications, developing an activity plan, and monitoring weight. Additionally, the Health Belief Model directs the nurse to inquire about the patient's view of negative aspects of these self-management activities [34].

Thus, after assessing the patient using scales such as those developed and tested by Bennett and colleagues [35, 29] or the Health Belief Model itself, it is possible to identify key issues for the patient and then develop an individually suited education plan.

Theory of reasoned action

In 1980, Ajzen and Fishbein [36] developed a theory to explain human behavior that is under voluntary control[30]. Underpinning this particular theory is the interaction between two major influences: personal beliefs about a particular behavior and the individual's perception of what significant others will think of their behavior [30]. These influences combine to form an intention for the individual to behave in a certain manner [37] and this intention is predicative of the health behavior [38]. The theory maintains that behavior is determined by intention and that the intentions of the individual are determined by personal attitude and social norms. [38]. The theory has also been further developed by the authors [36] to include perceived behavioral control as a third influence on behavioral intentions [30], identifying that a person's intentions will be more significant if they perceive that they have personal control over a behavior [30]. Sheeran and colleagues [39] further outline that intentions are predicted by three key factors:

- Attitudes: the attitudes that an individual may have toward a particular behavior.

- Subjective norms: an individual's perception of the social pressure from others to perform a particular behavior or not [39].
- Perceived behavioral control: an individual's perception of their own ability to perform the behavior.

Sheeran and colleagues [39] further propose that:

> The more positive people's attitudes and subjective norms are regarding a behaviour, and the greater their perceived behavioural control, the stronger people's intentions to perform the behaviour will be. Similarly, the stronger people's intentions, and the greater their perceived behavioural control the more likely it is that people will perform the behaviour [39].

The theory "predicts that a person is most likely to intend to adopt, maintain or change a behavior if they believe the behavior will benefit their health, is socially desirable and feels social pressure to behave in that way" [30].

Application of the theory to clinical practice research

A good example of the utilization of the Theory of Reasoned Action to improve the management of a chronic condition has been reported by Miller and colleagues [38]. This theory was applied in the context of improving compliance (sic) behaviors of hypertensive patients. They hypothesized that application of the model to outpatient instructions given to 56 newly diagnosed hypertensive patients would affect the compliance behavior of the prescriptions for diet, smoking, activity, and stress and medication within six months of implementing the study intervention [38]. The results from the study, although not controlled, indicated that the intervention was sufficient to affect the prescribed behaviors of diet, smoking, activity, and stress but not medication [38]. The application of this theory to chronic angina pectoris (as shown in Figure 6.4) demonstrates the main concepts underlying this theory and its potential role in symptom management and risk factor reduction in the setting of chronic cardiac care.

Social cognitive theory and social learning theory

Social Learning theory and Social Cognitive theory are closely related. Social Cognitive theory is considered to have progressed from Social Learning theory over the past 50 years due to the contributions of several researchers in the field, notably that of Bandura [40–42]. The Social Learning theory as proposed by Bandura [40] postulates that:

> ...most learning occurs by modelling rather than trial and error and that the more positive consequences of a behaviour change, the more likely people are to engage in it... [37].

Within this theory, a differentiation is made between the individual's belief in the outcome of the behavior and their own ability to perform specific behaviors in particular situations, with both concepts being vital to behavior change as

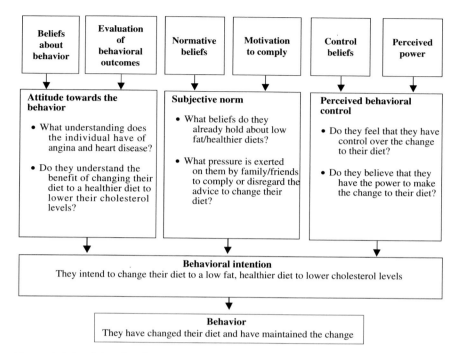

Figure 6.4 Applying the theory of reasoned action model – chronic angina pectoris. (Adapted from the original [30].)

outlined by Bandura [37]. Another key concept of the theory is both the internal and external loci of control, Baum outlines this concept:

> . . .internal locus of control where people believe they are responsible for their own health, and external locus of control where people see their health as being influenced primarily by outside forces. . . [37].

The concept of the external and internal locus of control is a fundamental aspect of health psychology. If the individual "owns" their own health and feels that they can do something to improve their health and that their actions can also harm their health, they are likely to adapt behaviors which lend to improving their health, rather than relying on external factors such as hospitals, doctors, etc. to improve their health for them. This concept once again relates to self-efficacy of the individual in relation to their health and well being.

A clinical study of the efficacy of the social learning theory

The MULTIFIT study [43] is an example of the application of the theory to the management of CHF. The MULTIFIT program is a physician-supervised, nurse-mediated, home-based system for CHF management based on the implantation of consensus guidelines for pharmacologic and dietary therapy with the aim to improve pharmacologic and dietary compliance and monitor clinical status [43]. It was demonstrated that for the 51 heart failure patients enroled in the study, the behavioral intervention, based on social learning theory as set out by Bandura [41] improved compliance to both pharmacologic and dietary therapy, improved self-management skills including self-monitoring of disease, and body weight [43]. The intervention utilized in the study included an initial session between the patient and nurse manager, whereby the patient was educated on their disease state, the role of sodium restriction and pharmacologic therapy and warning signs of CHF progression and behavioral techniques for improving compliance to both pharmacologic and dietary therapies [43]. This initial session was followed up by nurse-initiated telephone follow-up weekly for the ensuing six weeks [43]. Chapter 3 provides a more detailed overview of the MULTIFIT concept.

Transtheoretical model – stages of change

Developed by Prochaska and DiClimente [44] to represent the psychosocial process of smoking cessation, the model outlines discrete stages over which behavior may be changed. These stages are believed to occur whether the change occurs within or outside of a formal treatment process [45]. The five stages of the model include:

1 precontemplation (no intention to change behavior)
2 contemplation (thinking about the change)
3 preparation (commitment to change their behavior)
4 action (behavior changed successfully)
5 maintenance (behavior successfully maintained long-term) [45].

Since the model's development in the early 1980s, the model has been interpreted as having more or less than the current five accepted stages. Although the theory is outlined in succinct steps, the manner in which individuals may progress through the process is variable, with some going backwards and forwards throughout the process, rather than following straightforward through the steps [46]; this, however, has been debated by some along with the thought that the stages are not as discrete as they may appear, as discussed in Littell and Girvin's [45] critique of the model.

Application of the model in clinical setting and studies

This particular model has been extensively applied to the study and treatment of negative behaviors such as narcotic addiction and smoking, and in some instances positive behavior such as the use of sunscreen and mammograms [45,47]. By identifying the stage at which the individual is at, an appropriate intervention may be utilized to facilitate progression through the stages [47].

Sneed and Paul [48] studied CHF patient's stage of readiness for six lifestyle and health behaviors important in optimizing related health outcomes (e.g. reducing sodium intake, avoiding excess fluid intake, alcohol, and tobacco, and undertaking regular exercise and weight control). The mail survey of 250 CHF patients determined the differences in the signs and symptoms of the syndrome, self-reported knowledge of their condition along with self-reported behavior of whether an action had been undertaken or not [48]. This pilot study of the application of the model to CHF reported that "use of the stage of change tool to assess stage of readiness to make lifestyle changes may not work well in patients with heart failure": attributing this finding to the number and complexity of the changes required by the patient with CHF [48]. As such, although study participants "thought they were consistently adhering to recommended guidelines for changes in lifestyle, actual reported behaviors did not always support this evaluation" [48].

Dunbar and colleague's [34] interpretation of the application of the model to optimize education of CHF patients highlights the relationship between assessment of the stage the individual is at and the corresponding intervention:

> By assessing stage of change regarding a particular behavior or a lifestyle pattern and determining whether the patient has experience with attempting the change, the nurse can determine which interventions might be most effective in managing the heart failure. The specific motivational interventions vary by stage of change [34].

They then highlight that not only can the intervention include education but also rewards:

> ...interventions can include setting up a personal reward system, seeking the help of family members, and using a self-administered pep talk to focus on the positive aspects of what the patient is doing for his or her overall health [34].

Despite the findings of a study undertaken by Sneed and Paul [48], suggesting that the model may not be suitable for CHF patients, there are aspects of CHF management that represent natural targets in this regard (e.g. regulation of sodium intake) – see Figure 6.5.

Dorothea Orem's general nursing theory

Orem's General Theory of Nursing [49] is also considered in this chapter due to the potential reader base of the book. Dorothea Orem initiated the theory in the 1950s and was first published during the 1970s, with continual development of the theory over the proceeding years [50]. There are some key concepts of Orem's theory, which are outlined to provide an overview of the main concepts of the theory.

Self-care deficit nursing theory

Self-care is defined by Orem as "the practice of activities that the individuals initiate and perform on their own behalf in maintaining life, healthy functioning, personal development, and well-being" [51]. The theory focusses on the action capabilities of individuals and their demands for self-care [52]. The key concepts of this theory, adapted from the work of Orem [51] and published by Jaarsma [52], are outlined below:

- *Therapeutic self-care demand.* Represents the total activities that should be performed to maintain self-care [51].
- *Self-care agency.* Is required in order to engage in effective self-care.

Stage of change	Underlying process	Patient education
1 Pre-contemplation	Patient may be unaware of the relationship between sodium intake and heart failure symptoms.	Educate patient about chronic heart failure and the purpose of reducing sodium intake.
2 Contemplation	Patient is considering and reflecting on what they know about their condition and what role their diet plays in how they feel.	Discussion with patient about the benefit of reducing their sodium intake.
3 Preparation	Patient is considering changing habit, and is questioning how they might do so.	Assists patient with how they will manage reducing sodium intake and outlines potential barriers.
4 Action	Patient begins to reduce sodium intake, and may continue doing so in the short term.	A plan is formulated to enable the patient to enjoy meals and eating out but whilst maintaining their sodium restriction.
5 Maintenance	Patient has maintained lower sodium consumption in long term	Follow-up with the patient to see how they are managing the restriction and continue motivation.

Figure 6.5 Applying the stages of change model: management of sodium intake in CHF. (Adapted from the original [30].)

- *Self-care deficit.* When the individual's capabilities are inadequate to meet the therapeutic self-care demand, thus nursing care may be required [51,52].

For the latter to occur, three types of capabilities are necessary.

1 The ability to determine what needs to be done to regulate health and well being.

2 The ability to judge and decide what to do from the information obtained.

3 The ability to actually perform self-care actions once the knowledge is obtained and the decision to act has been made [51,52].

To begin a program addressing and encouraging self-care, the individual must be assessed for their therapeutic self-care demand, their self-care agency must be estimated, and the existence or potential for self-care deficits should be determined [52]. Jaarsma applied Orem's theories to the management of CHF, reporting at the time of her studies that "there is no known well-defined or structured program available that can be used to enhance heart failure patients' abilities to engage in self-care" [52].

Clinical research application of Orem's general theory of nursing

Jaarsma developed a supportive-educative program of care using Orem's General Theory of Nursing (specifically the Self-care Deficit Nursing Theory) for patients with CHF based on the premise that individuals effectively engaged in self-care do not require nursing care and thus will not require hospitalization [52]. The effects of such a program on self-care agency, prevention of readmission and quality of life was tested in a randomized controlled trial. In the study, 128 patients were randomly assigned to receive either "care-as-usual" or the "supportive-educative intervention". The intervention involved an "intensive, systematized and planned education by a study nurse about the consequences of heart failure on daily life," which included on average of four visits within hospital, one telephone call and one home visit by the study nurse [52]. From this study findings on the self-care behavior, resource utilization, and quality of life were reported. The findings of the study report that the effect of the supportive education intervention on heart failure-related self-care behavior was best observed within one month following discharge from hospital. Whilst both groups demonstrated improved self-care behavior within the first month, and a decline over time, those in the intervention group were more compliant (sic) with the prescribed self-care behaviors at three and nine months following discharge [52].

6.5 Summary

Considering all the evidence discussed and presented in this chapter regarding the role of education in improving and maintaining patient self-management in chronic cardiac conditions that is imperative to their success, it is important that the health care professional who facilitates patient education is equipped with the knowledge of how to present the strategies of self-management to a diverse and usually elderly population, with a range of chronic disease states.

References

1 Bodenheimer T, Lorig K, Holman H, et al. Patient self-management of chronic disease in primary care. *JAMA* 2002; **288**(19):2469–2475.

2 Lorig K. Chronic disease self-management: a model for tertiary intervention. *Am Behav Sci* 1996; **39**(6):676–683.

3 Bandura A. The anatomy of stages of change. *Am J Health Promot* 1997; **12**(1):8–10.

4 Levenson JW, McCarthy EP, Lynn J, et al. The last six months of life for patients with congestive heart failure. *J Am Geriatr Soc* 2000; **48**:S101–S109.

5 Krumholz HM, Phillips RS, Hamel MB, et al. Resuscitation preferences among patients with severe congestive heart failure: results from the SUPPORT project. *Circulation* 1998; **98**:648–655.

6 Koenig HG. Depression in hospitalized older patients with congestive heart failure. *Gen Hosp Psych* 1998; **20**: 29–43.

7 Freedland KE, Carney RM, Rich MW, et al. Depression in elderly patients with congestive heart failure. *Geriatr Psych* 1991; **24**:59–71.

8 Moore RK, Groves D, Bateson S, et al. Health related quality of life of patients with refractory angina before and one year after enrolment onto a refractory angina program *Eur J Pain* 2005;**9**(3):305–310.

9 Mast BT, Yochim B, MacNeill SE, et al. Risk factors for geriatric depression: the importance of executive functioning within the vascular depression hypothesis. *J Gerontol A Biol Sci Med Sci* 2004; **59**:1290–1294.

10 Luttik M, Jaarsma T, Van Veldhuisen DJ. Quality of life of caregivers is worse compared to patients with congestive heart failure. *Eur Heart J* 2003; **24**:64.

11 Murberg TA, Bru E, Aarsland T, *et al.* Functional status and depression among men and women with congestive heart failure. *Int J Psychiatry Med* 1998; **28**:273–291.

12 Evangelista LS, Kagawa-Singer M, Dracup K. Gender differences in health perceptions and meaning in persons living with heart failure. *Heart Lung* 2001; **30**(3):167–176.

13 Leventhal MJE, Reigel B, Carlson B, et al. Negiotating compliance in heart failure: Remaining issues and questions. *Eur J Cardiovasc Nurs* 2005; (E-pub May 11): In press.

14 Jennings B, Callahan D, Caplan AL. Ethical challenges of chronic illness. *Hasting Cent Rep* 1988; **18**(1):S1–S16.

15 Sabaté E. Adherence to long-term therapies: evidence for action. Geneva: World Health Organisation, 2003.

16 Hughes CM. Medication non-adherence in the elderly: how big is the problem? *Drugs Aging* 2004; **21**(12):793–811.

17 Taborski U, Muller-Berghaus G. State-of-the-art patient self-management for control of oral anticoagulation. *Semin Thromb Hemost* 1999; **25**:43–48.

18 White RH, McCurdy SA, Von Marensdorff H, et al. Home prothrombin time monitoring after the initiation of warfarin therapy: a randomised, prospective study. *Ann Intern Med* 1989; **11**:730–736.

19 Anderson DR, Harrison L, Hirsh J. Evaluation of portable prothrombin time monitor for home use by patients who require long-term oral anticoagulant therapy. *Arch Intern Med* 1993; **153**:1441–1447.

20 Ansell JE, Patel N, Ostrovsky D, et al. Long-term patient self-management of oral anticoagulation. *Arch Intern Med* 1995; **155**:2185–2189.

21 Eldor A, Schwartz J. Self-management of oral anticoagulants with a whole blood prothrombin-time monitor in elderly patients with atrial fibrillation. *Pathophysiol Haemost Thromb* 2002; **32**:99–106.

22 Monane M, Bohn RL, Gurwitz JH, et al. Non-compliance with congestive heart failure therapy in the elderly. *Arch Intern Med* 1994; **154**(4):433–437.

23 Cline CM, Bjorck-Linne AK, Israelsson BY, et al. Non-compliance and knowledge of prescribed medication in elderly patients with heart failure. *Eur J Heart Fail* 1999; **1**:145–9.

24 Bochachick P, Burke LE, Sereika S, et al. Adherence to angiotensin-converting enzyme inhibitor therapy for heart failure. *Prog Cardiovasc Nurse* 2002; **17**:(4)160–166.

25 Ni H, Nauman D, Burgess D, et al. Factors influencing knowledge of and adherence to self-care among patients with heart failure. *Arch Intern Med* 1999; **159**:(14)1613–1619.

26 Stewart S, Pearson S. Uncovering a multitude of sins: medication management in the home post acute hospitalisation among the chronically ill. *Aust NZ J Med* 1999; **29**:220–227

27 MacKay I, Stewart S. Optimising the day to day management of the patient with chronic heart failure. In: Stewart S, Blue L, eds., *Improving Outcomes in Chronic Heart*

Failure: specialist nurse intervention from research to practice. London: BMJ Publishing Group, 2004.

28 Becker MH. The health belief model and personal health behaviour. *Health Educ Monogr* 1974; **2**(4):324–508.

29 Bennett SJ, Perkins SM, Lane KA, et al. Reliability and validity of the compliance belief scales among patients with heart failure. *Heart and Lung* 2001; **30**(3):177–185.

30 Nutbeam D, Harris E. *Theory in a Nutshell: a practical guide to health promotion theories,* 2nd edn. Sydney, Australia: McGraw-Hill, 2004.

31 Janz NK, Becker MH. The health belief model: a decade later. *Health Educ Q* 1984; **11**:1–47.

32 Champion V. Beliefs about breast cancer and mammography by behavioural stage. *Onc Nurs Forum* 1994; **21**:1009–1014.

33 Redeker NS. Health beliefs and adherence in chronic illness. *Image* 1988; **20**:31–35.

34 Dunbar SB, Jacobson LH, Deaton C. Heart failure: strategies to enhance patient self-management. *AACN Clinical Issues* 1998; **9**(2):244–256.

35 Bennett SJ, Milgrom JB, Champion V, et al. Beliefs about medication and dietary compliance in people with heart failure: an instrument development study. *Heart and Lung* 1997; **26**:273–279.

36 Ajzen I, Fishbein M. *Understanding Attitudes and Predicting Social Behaviour.* Englewood Cliffs, NJ: Prentice Hall, 1980.

37 Baum F. *The New Public Health: an Australian perspective.* South Melbourne: Oxford University Press, 1998.

38 Miller P, Wikoff R, Hiatt A. Fishbein's model of reasoned action and compliance behaviour of hypertensive patients. *Nurs Res* 1992; **41**(2):104–109.

39 Sheeran P, Conner M, Norman P. Can the theory of planned behaviour explain patterns of health behaviour change? *Health Psychol* 2001; **20**(1):12–19.

40 Bandura A. self-efficacy: toward a unifying theory of behavioral change. *Psychol Rev* 1977; **84**(2): 191–215.

41 Bandura A. *Social Foundations of Thought and Action: a social cognitive theory.* Englewood Cliffs, NJ: Prentice-Hall, 1986.

42 Bandura A, ed. *Self-efficacy in Changing Societies.* Cambridge: Cambridge University Press, 1995.

43 West JA, Miller NH, Parker KM, et al. A comprehensive management system for heart failure improves clinical outcomes and reduces medical resource utilisation. *Am J Cardiol* 1997; **79**:58–63.

44 Prochaska JO, DiClimente CC. Self change processes, self efficacy and decisional balance across five stages of smoking cessation. *Prog Clin Biol Res* 1984; **156**:131–140.

45 Littell JH, Girvin H. Stages of change: a critique. *Behav Modif* 2002; **26** (2):223–273.

46 Prochaska JO, DiClimente CC. Stages of change in the modification of problem behaviours. *Prog Behav Modif* 1992; **28**:183–218.

47 Ni Mhurchu C, Margetts BM, Speller VM. Applying the stages of change model to dietary change. *Nutr Rev* 1997; **55**(1):10–16.

48 Sneed NV, Paul SC. Readiness for behavioural changes in patients with heart failure. *Am J Crit Care* 2003; **12**(5):444.

49 Orem D. *Nursing: Concepts of Practice.* New York: McGraw-Hill, 1971.

50 Goodwin M. Is it feasible for the nursing division at St Vincent's Hospital to adopt Dorothea Orem's model of nursing? St Vincent's Nursing Monograph 1990: Selected Works. Accessed online 22 July 2005 at http://www.clininfo.health.nsw.gov.au/hospolic/stvincents/1990/a06.html
51 Orem DE. *Nursing: Concepts of Practice*, 5th edn. St Louis: Mosby, 1995.
52 Jaarsma T. *Heart Failure: Nurses Care*. Maastricht: Datawyse, 1998.

Section 4
Optimizing Chronic Cardiac Care

CHAPTER 7

Establishing a nurse-led program of chronic cardiac care

7.1 Introduction

The typically poor health outcomes associated with chronic cardiac disease described in Chapter 1 should come as no surprise to anyone given the progressive nature of cardiac dysfunction with age and the inherently complex interaction between the individual, their treatment, and the many components of the health care system within which they are managed. However, there is a clear sense that if we were to spend as much time generating therapeutic solutions as applying them, we would be able make substantive inroads into high cost and highly debilitating conditions, such as chronic cardiac disease. It is within this context that this chapter builds upon the extensive data and literature synthesized in previous chapters to build a framework for establishing a nurse-led program of chronic cardiac care.

7.2 Creating a strategic blueprint

As described in Chapter 5 (refer to Figure 5.1), once the need to optimize chronic cardiac care at the local, regional, or national level has been identified (and will be acted upon!) it is important for an expert panel to review the literature and the pattern of chronic cardiac disease to create a strategic blueprint that will be sensitive to the needs of affected individuals via a pragmatic application of the most cost-effective health care. As noted in Chapter 2, there is an inherent difficulty in applying the complex guidelines at the individual level. Similarly, there is also an inherent difficulty in applying these at the other end of the spectrum (i.e. at the whole service level). In some countries (e.g. the USA) there are difficulties in overcoming a fragmented health care system, while in other countries (e.g. Australia) there are difficulties in reaching a fragmented patient population. Figure 7.1 illustrates the fragmented nature of the Australian population via the distribution of patients with CHF with a large proportion living in rural and remote regions [1]. Clearly, there is no logic in "prescribing" the same form of nurse-led chronic cardiac care service (even if based on the same principles of care) for these two countries. In Australia, the need to reach those individuals with chronic cardiac

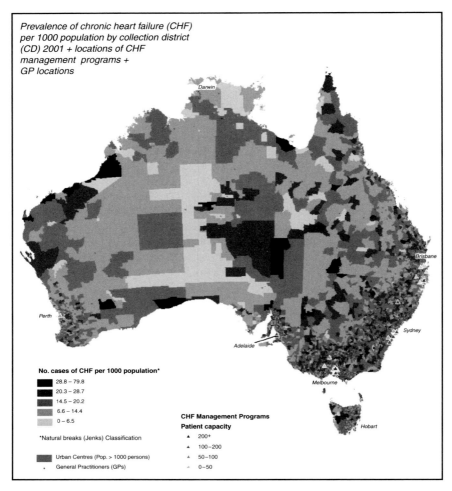

Figure 7.1 Distribution of CHF in Australia: the mismatch between supply and demand for primary care and specialist management programs in rural and remote regions. (Adapted from the original [1].)

disease distal to specialist centers of care, which requires the application of the type of remote technology/strategies outlined in Chapters 3 and 4, is clearly indicated.

As part of the critical processes outlined in Chapter 5, it is essential to outline the entire scope of service activity and its overall impact on health care costs and outcomes (both at the service and individual level). As described in a previous text specifically exploring the potential impact of a nurse-led, CHF management service in the UK, there are clear economic benefits to be derived from such a service [2]: these benefits are more than likely to extend to

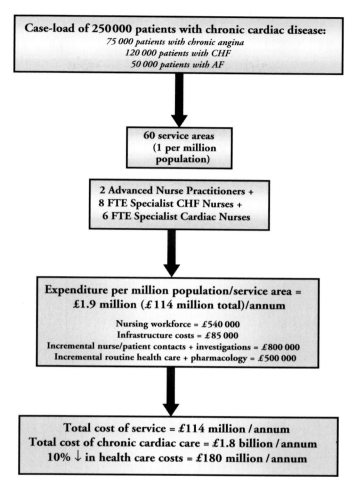

Figure 7.2 Potential cost profile (expenditure versus savings) of a UK-wide, nurse-led, chronic cardiac care service in the year 2000.

other Western developed countries [3]. In the absence of a similar economic analysis examining the wider impact of extending the framework of such a service to include the additional management of patients with chronic angina pectoris and AF, Figure 7.2, has used the same cost assumptions originally used to estimate the cost of a UK CHF service in the UK (total patient caseload of 120,000 per annum being managed at a cost of £70 million per annum), and used the key estimates outlined in Figures 1.14 and 1.19 to determine the cost of extending a combined service managing an additional 125,000 patients with chronic angina pectoris and AF; remembering that many patients with these conditions would have already been "captured" on the basis of concurrent CHF. Overall, this "ideal" service would cost approximately £120 million per annum to run. Although this represents an enormous sum, it only represents 6% of preexisting health care expenditure for these three key conditions. Like CHF, however, there is a substantial and preventable component of health care expenditure relating to angina pectoris and AF that, if even partially addressed (e.g. reducing the overall cost of health care expenditure by 10%), would derive significant cost-benefits; remembering that most strategies improve patient quality of life.

A figure similar to that of Figure 7.2 is essential, therefore, to outlining the scope of any proposed program or service, what resources it requires, and what is subsequently feasible in respect to the specifics of cardiac intervention and subsequent health outcomes.

7.3 A key role for the specialist cardiac nurse

Regardless of the form of service to be applied, it is reasonable to suggest that a typical ageing Western population with an ever-increasing burden of chronic cardiac disease be serviced in the following ways:

- A minimum of two nurse coordinators of chronic cardiac care per 1 million population.
- A minimum of eight full-time equivalent specialist CHF nurses to effectively manage CHF patients.
- Four to six appropriately trained cardiac nurses to manage patients with chronic angina pectoris and AF.

Consistent with the strategic role of chronic cardiac care beyond traditional cardiac rehabilitation (as outlined in Chapter 3), it is important to note that the provision of a such a service should not replace the critical role of cardiac rehabilitation; unfortunately, the short-sighted temptation by health care administrators to divert vital resources and personnel from cardiac rehabilitation to CHF care has been a widespread phenomenon.

Nurse practitioners versus specialist clinical nurse. A key question of course is what type of skill/knowledge mix is required to apply effective chronic cardiac care? There has been an ongoing international debate in respect to the relative merits of introducing advanced nurse practitioners to improve health outcomes. The International Council of Nurses defines a nurse practitioner as "a registered nurse who has acquired the expert knowledge base, complex decision-making skills and clinical competencies for extended practice, the characteristics of which are shaped by the context and/or country in which s/he is credentialed to practice". [4]

The nurse practitioner movement began in the USA in the 1960s. The first nurse practitioner program was developed by Silver and Ford in 1965 and operated at the University of Colorado (1967). Initially developed due to a shortage of primary care doctors in disadvantaged communities, the nurse practitioner role soon proved beneficial in the provision of effective, safe, and accessible health care [5,6]. Consequently, nurse practitioners were gradually accepted into the mainstream of health care services [7], such that by 1997, over 42,000 nurses were registered as nurse practitioners in the USA [1]. In the USA, nurse practitioners are credentialed in each state rather than nationally, resulting in variability in educational qualifications, role responsibilities, and level of autonomy and authority. Nurse practitioners have legislative authority to prescribe in 49 states of the USA and have been granted reimbursement by Medicare [8].

One of the confusing issues surrounding the nurse practitioner role is the use of nomenclature. In the USA, there are a variety of advanced practice roles; however, the boundaries between each role have become blurred. The American Nurses Association defines advanced nursing practice as a clinical role that requires a graduate degree in nursing. Nurse practitioners in clinical roles function in a multidisciplinary environment requiring a high level of autonomy and expert knowledge and skills, including comprehensive patient assessment, diagnosis, and treatment of potential health problems. In the UK, the nurse practitioner role was introduced in the early 1980s [9]. As in the USA, the nurse practitioner role in the UK was developed due to a shortage of doctors and a need to improve accessibility to health services in disadvantaged communities [10].

On an international basis, there is confusion in respect to the definition and role of the clinical nurse specialist and the advanced nurse practitioner. Both roles fall under the advanced practice umbrella, and advanced assessment skills, competencies, and knowledge are similar in both roles. In Australia there is a clearer boundary between nurse practitioners and clinical nurse specialists due the extension of practice of nurse practitioners in respect to prescribing, writing referrals and, in some States, admitting privileges. In the UK, a clinical nurse specialist is generally considered to be a nurse with in-depth specialist knowledge concerning a specific group of patients, while a nurse practitioner has been described as an autonomous doctor substitution role. In both countries, the *majority* of specialist CHF nurses operate within the boundaries associated with clinical nurse specialists. Pending the resolution of an ongoing international debate and, based on the practical realities of creating an effective workforce to optimize chronic cardiac care, it is prudent to suggest that there should be a *minimum* of two advanced nurse practitioners to service a population area of one million people to coordinate effective chronic cardiac care. Consistent with the creation of a workforce of specialist CHF nurses in many countries, the majority of which practice within the boundaries usually associated with that reserved for the "specialist clinical nurses", it is reasonable to suggest that the majority of nurses who would apply chronic cardiac care would have the following core characteristics:

- Professionally qualified as a nurse (for example, Registered Nurse).
- At least five years experience overall.
- At least two years of recent cardiology experience.
- Excellent communication skills.
- Experience in working in an autonomous position.
- A proven ability to work effectively in a multidisciplinary setting.
- Some computing skills.

Ideally, they would also have the following characteristics (some of which could be addressed by a formal training program):
- Previous community-based nursing experience.
- Specific expertise (skills and knowledge-base) in assessing, preventing, and managing cardiovascular risk factors.
- Specific expertise (skills and knowledge-base) in managing patients with CHF, chronic angina pectoris, AF and other common disease states (e.g. diabetes).
- Postbasic qualifications (for example, Critical Care Certificate) and/or higher nursing qualifications (Masters level).
- Experience in research and/or auditing.
- Advanced information technology skills.

Based on the strategic blueprint outlined in Figure 7.2, it would be reasonable to recruit and/or train a minimum of 12–14 specialist cardiac nurses to service a population of one million to provide specialist chronic cardiac care with key support from two or more advanced nurse practitioners. Clearly, any changes in this ratio will have an impact on the cost of implementing a program or service. Alternatively, advanced nurse practitioners may be expected to deliver more cost-benefits overall.

7.4 Screening and recruitment

While selecting and training a specialized workforce of nurses with an appropriate mix of expert knowledge and clinical skills is an important part of the process of building a nurse-led program (or service) of chronic cardiac care, it is *essential* to select the right patients with chronic cardiac disease for specialist intervention. In creating a strategic blueprint, an expert panel (particularly one with limited resources) will inevitably want to target those who would most benefit from the new created program/service.

Principles of selecting high-risk patients

In today's environment of "economic rationalism" and "evidence-based" health care there is an overwhelming tendency to overanalyze and micromanage health care to ensure that the appropriate health outcomes relative to investment of expertise and resources are obtained. Certainly, the contents of this book are largely a reflection of the need to justify and explain where and how health dollars are being used in otherwise inefficient health care systems. Hopefully, Chapter 1 has provided more than enough evidence to suggest that a significant proportion of individuals suffering from chronic cardiac disease not only suffer from disabling symptoms, but also impose a significant and increasing burden on already stressed health care systems. Clearly, however, a selection of individuals most at risk of poor health outcomes is mandated by limited health care resources. Unfortunately, this means that the most "proactive" of programs that systematically screen the community for those suffering from symptomatic cardiac disease are unlikely to be funded: particularly when there is a dearth of evidence to support such an initiative. Similarly, there is still a lack of definitive evidence to suggest that screening, and subsequently managing, patients who are being routinely managed via a general practitioner/primary care physician is likely to yield to a range of better health outcomes.

The major focus of screening for patients who would benefit from specialist nurse-led, chronic cardiac care at this stage, therefore, should still reside within the *hospital environment*. There are a number of inherent advantages to establishing a program of care within such a setting in order to screen and enroll suitable patients via inpatient and outpatient contacts:

- As indicated in Chapter 2, all three of the most common chronic cardiac disease states require advanced therapeutics based on definitive investigations and specialist opinion (e.g. echocardiography, coronary angiogram, and electrophysiologic studies).
- Optimal chronic cardiac care requires a multidisciplinary approach.
- The most successful programs have expert leadership/sponsorship (e.g. a cardiologist or specialist physician).
- Individuals who require hospital care (even if for more definitive investigation and treatment, and particularly for emergency treatment) represent a "high risk" patient group. Efforts to screen for, and subsequently find, eligible patients is likely to be much easier compared to "population" or "primary care screening" programs.

The following section details specific inclusion criteria that can be used to select inherently "high-risk" patients with chronic cardiac disease: consistent with the need to develop a program that is strategically relevant to the needs of the local population and health care system, such inclusion criteria should be individually formulated and adapted to each distinct service area. Before outlining these specific criteria, it is important to note a natural tendency to generate overcomplicated inclusion and exclusion criteria. Although there is a need to select patients who would most benefit from effective chronic cardiac care (and therefore derive the greatest cost savings), it is worth noting that the use of relatively simple criteria can delineate between high- and low-risk patients in the hospital context. For example, Figure 7.3 compares the long-term event-free survival curves of a large cohort of hospitalized patients who were prospectively designated as high- or low-risk on the following basis:

- Age $\geq$ 60 years.
- Prescription of $\geq$ 2 medications.
- Unplanned admission within preceding six months.
- Living alone and/or possessing limited English language skills.

Inclusion and exclusion criteria

In order to select appropriate patients to be managed in an evidence-based manner and to control patient throughput, strict but still widely applicable inclusion criteria have to be utilized. When combined, the following criteria are likely to recruit a core group of patients with chronic cardiac disease who

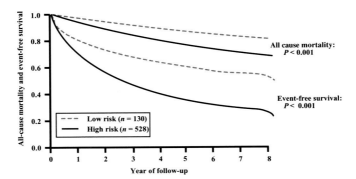

Figure 7.3 Comparison of long-term health outcomes in "low" versus "high risk" chronically ill patients discharged from acute hospital care. (Adapted from the original report/data [11].

would most benefit from optimal management and provide the greatest cost-benefits via better health outcomes.

Chronic angina pectoris. This will most likely (but not exclusively) be the youngest group of patients. An acute coronary syndrome (fatal or otherwise) is the most common first manifestation of heart disease that brings an individual to the attention of the health care system. Many patients will be discharged from definitive medical/surgical care without chronic symptoms indicative of angina pectoris angina. The following criteria are likely to identify those most in need of specialist management:

> Patients admitted to participating hospitals or managed on an outpatient basis, will be asked to participate if they are aged ≥45 years, reside in their own home, have coronary artery disease confirmed by coronary angiography, are in and require chronic antianginal therapy (other than episodic sublingual nitrate therapy) for chronic angina pectoris indicative of Canadian Heart Class II, III or IV.

Chronic heart failure. In all probability this group of patients will form the largest component of a "hybrid" chronic cardiac care service. The majority of patients will be aged >65 years with a mean age of 75 years. Experience suggests that if the following criteria are used to select patients via systematic screening of all inpatient activity (not necessarily confined to a specialist cardiology unit) at a reasonably sized acute care hospital (e.g. >250 beds), a rapid patient caseload will be established:

> Patients admitted to participating hospitals will be offered specialist management if they are aged ≥55 years, to be discharged to home, have an underlying diagnosis of CHF with related persistent moderate to severe symptoms and a history of ≥1 admission for acute heart failure.

The majority of studies included in the meta-analyses outlined in Chapter 4 have included patients on the basis of chronic symptomatic CHF associated with both impaired and preserved (so-called diastolic failure) left ventricular function. It is advisable, therefore, to determine the presence of moderate-severe CHF based on the recently updated ESC guidelines outlined in Chapter 2, with confirmation (via echocardiography or radionuclide ventriculography) of impaired left ventricular systolic (definition = left ventricular ejection fraction [LVEF] ≤45%) *OR* preserved left ventricular systolic function (LVEF >45% and evidence of abnormal LV relaxation/filling/distensibility indices on cardiac catheterization *or* echocardiographic concentric LV without wall motion abnormalities). Assessment of persistent functional impairment/symptoms should be based on NYHA Class II, III, or IV status. Acute heart failure should be confirmed on the basis of pulmonary congestion/ edema on chest radiography, with a clinical syndrome of acute dyspnoea at rest.

Chronic atrial fibrillation. As this condition typically appear at the end of the chronic cardiac disease spectrum, it is likely that many (but not all) patients with chronic AF will already have underlying angina and/or CHF. They are also likely to be older than the two previous patient cohorts. Regardless of the overlap, the following criteria, when applied on the same basis as that of CHF, are likely to yield a significant number of patients requiring specialist management:

> Patients admitted to participating hospitals or managed on an outpatient basis, will be asked to participate if they are aged ≥ 45 years, reside in their own home and require *chronic* antiarrhythmic or anticoagulation therapy for chronic AF (persistent or permanent).

The recent ACC/AHA/ESC guidelines define chronic forms of AF as follows:
- Persistent AF: is not self-terminating and may require treatment in the form of chemical or electrical cardioversion (so called "rhythm control" management): left untreated, episodes may last longer than seven days and may be recurrent in nature.
- Permanent AF: may take the form of paroxysmal or persistent AF; however, either due to a clinical decision to limit the underlying ventricular rate (so-called "rate control" management) or due to failed cardioversion, patients require chronic treatment.

A universal list of *exclusion criteria* can be applied in all three contexts:
- Unwilling to have additional specialist support.
- Significantly cognitive impairment determined by the abbreviated mini-mental test.
- Major communication problems.
- Other immediately life threatening illness (e.g. advanced malignancy).
- Living outside of the institutional/health care authority geographic area of responsibility.
- Discharged to long-term care (e.g. nursing home care).
- Attending day hospital facilities on a regular basis for medical management (e.g. a preestablished cardiac clinic that would obviate the need for additional management).
- Patient history of abusive behavior toward health care professionals.

If a patient does not *strictly* meet the inclusion criteria but they may still potentially benefit from more intensive management, their possible recruitment to the program/service may be negotiated.

Recruitment

In order to recruit eligible patients it is imperative that the specialist program/service and its inclusion/exclusion criteria are widely known. In many cases, patients will be recruited from specific areas within an acute care hospital (e.g. general medical and cardiology wards plus a specialist anticoagulation clinic). However, in many ways the most difficult process is identifying and "capturing" *all* eligible patients: patients often need to be identified without delay while in hospital and this requires that the multidisciplinary team involved in their care are aware of the existence and operational parameters of the chronic cardiac care service and how to access it. This requires a team approach within the hospital from which patients are recruited. While it is true that the specialist nurse is probably most qualified to screen all admitted patients, screening is a time-consuming process and, after completing a baseline assessment of all eligible patients, they would have little time to do anything else.

Clearly, therefore, there needs to be mechanisms by which eligible patients are identified and referred to the specialist nurse for possible intervention. Information about the program/service should be clearly displayed in all areas with a high concentration of potentially eligible patients. Due to the almost universal turnover of staff in large organizations, it is important to raise the profile of the program/service on a regular basis to avoid appropriate patients being missed. Key strategies in this regard are:

- Educational talks to nursing staff.
- Presentations at grand rounds.
- Regular visits to inpatient and outpatient units.
- Employing a dedicated recruitment officer.

7.5 Principles of effective chronic cardiac care

As extensively described in Chapter 2, there is a wealth of effective therapies and expert opinion to guide the management of all three of the most common manifestations of chronic cardiac disease. Rather than rewrite these guidelines, particularly as the latest iterations now explicitly acknowledge the role of multidisciplinary management and therapeutics beyond pharmacotherapy and devices, we strongly suggest that this section be regarded as a practical framework for applying the evidence in patients with chronic cardiac disease. As the practical experience of chronic cardiac care increases overall, (for a detailed guide to the management of CHF refer to *Improving Outcomes in Chronic Heart Failure: Specialist Nurse Intervention from Research to Practice* [12]), texts of this type will be able to provide much more definitive detail of the practical application and impact of specific strategies relating to chronic angina pectoris and AF.

Baseline assessment

Before actively managing a patient who agrees to be specially managed, it is imperative that an initial, comprehensive profile of the patient (and family/carers if appropriate) and their past health care utilization and management be compiled. Using a review of the patient's medical records, personal interviews with the patient and/or treating physician, the following baseline data should collected for each patient:

- *Demographic profile.* Age, sex, marital status, social support, income, education, and ethnicity.
- *Past history.* Risk factor profile, contributory conditions, and pattern of health care utilization.
- *Clinical status.* Type, presumed cause and duration of chronic angina, CHF and/or AF, type of nonpharmacologic treatment, body mass index, blood counts (including Hb level), electrolytes, thyroid/renal/hepatic function, past and concurrent cardiac and noncardiac disease states (e.g. Charlson Index calculated [13]) and all echocardiographic, coronary angiography and electrophysiological data.
- *Medical/Surgical.* All therapy relative to expert guidelines.
- *Functional/general health status.* Six-minute walk test with monitoring of ventricular response, Mini-Mental test [14] and a suitable health-related quality of life instrument (e.g. the EQ-5D [15], SF-36 [16] or Minnesota Living with Heart Failure Survey) [17].

The most effective services are supported by advanced information technology. A dedicated data set with entry of baseline data and comprehensive records relating to subsequent patient contacts, nonfatal morbid events and key health outcomes (see auditing section below) with linkage to all inpatient, outpatient, and investigational data sets is extremely useful both at the individual and service levels. The letters generated are structured in accordance with good communication guidelines.

Individualized patient follow-up and support

One of the key aims of effective chronic cardiac management is to provide tailored management to meet the individual's needs in accordance with the program/service's therapeutic guidelines/protocols. In most nurse-led initiatives the specialist cardiac nurse will be ultimately responsible for (even if not initiating or prescribing) the following:

- Continued adjustment and optimization of medical and nonpharmacological therapy where indicated.
- Monitoring the patient's cardiac risk, clinical status, and results of specific investigations: particularly if there is evidence of clinical instability and deteriorating symptoms, or if changes to the therapeutic regimen have been made.

Naturally this encompasses a broad scope of clinical practice and activity. If one were to accept an optimal workload of 200–250 CHF patients *or* 275 to 325 patients with other forms of chronic heart disease per specialist cardiac nurse/annum, there is a clear need to work strategically to maximise patient contacts. As noted in Chapter 6, a previously underrecognized resource within the health care system is the person with the most to gain from effective management – the patient! It is within this context that the every effort should be made, after assessing each patient's ability to self-care that they be encouraged to take a proactive role in their health and health management. As such, effective patient preparations is not just a matter of simply providing information, but allowing them to develop capacity to observe themselves, make sensible judgments, feel confident, and recognize desired outcomes [18]. Within this context, Table 7.1 (adapted from the original) shows the complexity of self-care behaviors relating to the management of CHF: similar tables could be quite simply constructed in respect to modifiable risk factors and the specific management of chronic angina pectoris and AF.

Practical research undertaken by Riegel and colleagues in the setting of CHF demonstrate the potential for promoting self-care behaviors: asserting that the self-care decision making is a complex process [19]. They define self-care in this setting as an active cognitive process and proposed a five-stage model that is derived from a naturalistic decision making process. In this model, self-management is perceived to be a component of self-care. Stage 1 acknowledges the choice of behaviors that are adopted to maintain physiologic stability and is termed "self-care maintenance". Recording a daily weight, restricting sodium intake, exercising regularly, maintaining a healthy body mass index, and getting annual inoculations against flu and pneumonia are typical self-care maintenance behaviors. A family member or carer may provide some external direction in self-care maintenance; for example; in recording the trend in daily weights. Stages 2, 3, 4, and 5 reflect "self-care management" [19,20]. These stages require patients to recognize changes in their health in order for them to respond to symptoms appropriately and evaluate the effectiveness of any remedies that have been initiated to lessen the symptom. Self-care is, therefore, a complex cognitive process that involves recognition of the symptom and appraisal of its importance, implementing an action or remedy, and evaluating its effectiveness [19,20].

Clearly, self-care activities do not represent a "panacea" in improving outcomes in chronic cardiac disease [21]: particularly given the advanced age and impaired cognitive function of many patients, in addition to a common lifelong adoption of a passive role in the presence of health authority figures. The inherent risk profile (including ability to self-care) and clinical status of each patient should determine the level of patient contacts and intervention as part of effective chronic cardiac care.

Assessment criteria and schedule of follow-up nurse contact

Regardless of their risk profile and clinical status, all patients (and their family and carers where appropriate) enrolled in chronic cardiac care program should be offered minimum specialist nurse-led contact comprising the following type of follow-up:

Table 7.1 Outline of common self-care activities in managing CHF. (Adapted from the original [18].)

Behavior	Key indicator of clinical status	Patient-initiated actions
Daily weight	• Sudden increase in weight of >1.5 kg • Increasing peripheral edema of feet, legs, abdomen	• Reduce fluid intake to 1.5 liters • Reduce sodium intake <2 g/day • Take an extra diuretic • Report symptoms • Take all medications as instructed by your doctor but consider taking an extra diuretic
Monitoring symptoms for worsening HF	• Worsening breathlessness, especially at night • Waking up through the night with cough and shortness of breath, sleeping on an increasing number of pillows • Reduced exercise capacity • Increased lethargy • Abdominal bloating and loss of appetite/nausea • Sudden weight loss of >2 kg, dry mouth, increased thirst and reduced urine output	• Sleep on extra pillows • Reduce fluid intake to 1.5 liters • Reduce sodium intake <2 g/day • Take all medications as instructed by your doctor but consider taking an extra diuretic • Pace yourself • Report symptoms • Temporarily cease fluid restriction and report symptoms
Regular exercise	• Reduced exercise capacity • Excessive tiredness/lethargy • Need for more rest periods • Increasing angina	• Plan your day and pace yourself (energy conservation and pacing) • Keep as active as possible but ask for help to attend with heavy activities • Discuss symptoms with your doctor/ physiotherapist

(Continued)

Table 7.1 *Continued*

Behavior	Key indicator of clinical status	Patient-initiated actions
Adhere to prescribed therapy	• Increased dizziness/postural hypotension, • Adverse effects of prescribed therapy (particularly if impairs social activities) • Occasionally missing medications • Confusion about medications due to polypharmacy • Forgetting to obtain repeat medications	• Understand your medications and spread out cardiac medications over the day • Discuss alternative times for taking medications • Use dossette box or daily reminders • Ask for clear written medication instructions to help in understanding your medications • Involve your pharmacist in solving medication problems • Make regular appointments with your doctor/cardiologist to review medications
Maintain optimal nutrition/weight	• Abnormal weight loss and muscle wastage • Persistent peripheral edema • Unable to loose excess weight	• Eat frequent, small, high calorific meals • Restrict dietary sodium intake • Reduce calorie and fat intake, exercise regularly • Discuss nutritional problems with a dietician
Annual flu/pneumococcal vaccinations	• Readmissions to hospital during winter months with congestive HF / chest infections	• Maintain regular follow-up with local doctor

• A home or specialist clinic visit within one week of an index hospital discharge or outpatient recruitment to comprehensively assess their baseline characteristics.
• A second home or specialist clinic visit after 1–4 weeks (substituted by telephone follow-up if too remote)
• A phone call at three months (substituted with home visit if no telephone)
• Immediate access to the program/service if they are readmitted to hospital or other serious morbid event

Based on the following three components of assessment, patients should be subject to a more prolonged and intensive program of follow-up:

1 *Cardiac risk profile.* Patients should be carefully assessed to determine if they have any modifiable cardiovascular risk factors that can potentially slow the progression of underlying cardiac disease.

2 *Symptomatic status.* Patients can be (arbitrarily) divided into those who are symptomfree and those in whom symptoms persist following hospital discharge. In both of these groups there will be patients who are either at "low" or "high" risk for future events such as unplanned readmission or even death without hospitalization.

3 *Appropriateness of treatment.* Regardless of an individual's symptoms, treatment will be either appropriate or inappropriate.

In combination with the above parameters, the likely outcome for individual patients and subsequent extent of surveillance and support can be further delineated on the basis of the overall risk profile of the patient (as opposed to specific risk factors for more cardiac events):

1 *Low-risk* patients are typically characterized by the following features:
- Knowledgeable about their condition and treatment.
- Adhere to prescribed pharmacological and nonpharmacological therapies.
- Receive adequate social support.
- Not in need of dramatic changes in their therapeutic management and/or demonstrate a clear ability to self-care (see above).

2 *High-risk* patients are typically characterized by the following features
- A poor understanding of their condition and its treatment.
- A history of recurrent admissions to hospital and/or a near-fatal event.
- Poor adhere to prescribed pharmacological and nonpharmacological therapies.
- Inadequate social support.
- Need for complex changes to treatment and/or poor self-care behaviors.

It should be noted that these are principles of assessment only and that ultimately, it is the expert judgement of the specialist cardiac nurse, in conjunction with the advice of the other health care professionals and the availability of resources (i.e. by considering current caseload demands) that determines the duration and intensity of follow-up. However, using the above criteria, it is possible to roughly categorize the needs of patients using the following groups and the intensity and frequency of care modulated accordingly.

Group 1 Patients: found to be clinically stable at the initial assessment

(A) Low risk and appropriately treated

For patients at low risk and appropriately treated regular home visiting is unlikely to have much benefit and telephone contact on an infrequent basis (for example, three monthly) is all that is required. These patients will be encouraged to make nonscheduled telephone contact should their condition deteriorate. These patients will therefore receive the "minimum service" unless their condition or risk profile subsequently changes. Their ability to self-care is both encouraged and supported.

(B) Low risk but inappropriately treated or presence of modifiable cardiovascular risk factor

In this group of patients the main aim is to optimize the patient's medication in accordance with the programs/service protocols and guidelines (i.e. based on those listed in Chapter 2). Patients may be assessed weekly (via home visit, clinic appointment, or telephone call) until their therapeutic regimen is appropriate and all their parameters (e.g. lipid profile or renal function) are stable. These patients are encouraged to make nonscheduled telephone contact should their condition deteriorate or they have trouble maintaining a low-risk profile (e.g. inability to maintain an exercise program alone and would prefer group activities of the same). Their ability to self-care is both encouraged and supported.

(C) High risk but appropriately treated

In high-risk, appropriately treated patients, intervention is aimed at improving the patient's understanding of their condition(s) and its treatment, and where indicated increasing social support. The patient may be assessed weekly until modifiable risk factors are fully addressed, in accordance with the patient's needs and wishes. Regular telephone calls may also be required until all modifiable issues are addressed. Patients will also be encouraged to make nonscheduled telephone contact should their condition deteriorate.

(D) High risk and inappropriately treated

The intervention in high-risk patients who are inappropriately treated is aimed at improving the patient's understanding of their condition(s) and its treatment; where indicated, increasing social support; and optimizing the patient's medication in accordance with the agreed medication guidelines. Active assessment and intervention may be undertaken on a weekly basis until the patient is compliant with an appropriate therapeutic regimen and modifiable risk factors have been fully addressed, in accordance with the patient's needs and wishes. Regular telephone calls may also be required until all modifiable issues are addressed. Patients will also be encouraged to make nonscheduled telephone contact should their condition deteriorate.

Group 2 Patients: clinically unstable or uncontrolled symptoms at the initial assessment
(A) Low risk and appropriately treated

One of the objectives of specialist nurse intervention in low-risk appropriately treated patients is, where possible, to adjust what is already considered to be appropriate therapy to improve the patient's clinical status and to minimize any adverse effects of treatment. This will involve application of the therapeutic guidelines and protocols with appropriate monitoring of any therapeutic changes (e.g. improved functional status). The patient *may* require a number of comprehensive assessments (via home or clinic visits whenever possible) if there is scope for symptoms to improve. *It must be acknowledged, however, that it may not be possible to resolve symptoms completely in all patients and therefore further adjustment of treatment may be inappropriate.* However, the patient is also likely to benefit from other components of this type of intervention. The second objective, therefore, is to provide additional support to individuals who remain symptomatic despite optimal therapy but who would, for example, benefit from psychological and/or, ultimately, palliative care support. On this basis, further interventions may be warranted, followed by regular telephone follow-up thereafter. Patients will also be encouraged to make nonscheduled telephone contact should their condition deteriorate.

(B) Low risk but inappropriately treated or presence of modifiable cardiovascular risk factors

The purpose of the intervention in this group of patients is to adjust their therapy to improve clinical status, minimize adverse effects and modify cardiovascular risk factors,: once again via application of the therapeutic guidelines and protocols with appropriate monitoring of any therapeutic changes (e.g. optimal lipid profile). Patients will require regular intervention until their symptoms/risk factor profile improves and the patient adheres to an appropriate regimen. Regular telephone calls may be required until appropriate therapy or clinical stability is achieved. *It may not be possible to resolve symptoms completely in all patients even after appropriate treatment is implemented.* Patients will also be encouraged to make nonscheduled telephone contact should their condition deteriorate.

(C) High risk but appropriately treated

The object of intervention in high-risk patients who are appropriately treated is to adjust therapy to improve symptoms and signs and to minimize the potential for adverse effects. As before, this will involve application of the therapeutic guidelines and protocols with appropriate monitoring of any therapeutic changes (e.g. improved functional status). Patients may increase surveillance contacts until symptoms have improved and risk factors are fully addressed in accordance with the patient's needs and wishes. Regular telephone contact should be maintained until all important issues are addressed. *It may not be possible to resolve symptoms completely in all patients.* Patients will also be encouraged to make nonscheduled telephone contact should their condition deteriorate.

(D) High risk and inappropriately treated or presence of modifiable cardiovascular risk factors

The object of intervention in inappropriately treated, high-risk patients is to adjust therapy to improve the patient's clinical status and minimize any adverse effects of treatment: as above, this will involve application of the therapeutic guidelines and protocols with appropriate monitoring of any therapeutic changes (e.g. improved functional status). Patients may require weekly home or clinic visits until they are adherent to an appropriate therapeutic regimen, their symptoms have improved, and modifiable risk factors have been fully addressed in accordance with the patient's needs and wishes. Regular telephone contact should be maintained until allimportant issues are addressed. *Once again, it should be remembered that it may not be possible to resolve symptoms completely in all patients.* Patients will also be encouraged to make nonscheduled telephone contact should their condition deteriorate.

Note: It is this group of patient who, potentially, would most benefit from the latest remote technologies to monitor clinical status and adherence to a therapeutic plan: particularly if they are unable (or unwilling) to be assessed in their own home or specialist clinic.

Summary of chronic cardiac care based on clinical status, modifiable risks and therapeutics

Table 7.2 is a theoretical schedule of a home-based chronic cardiac care program based on the above categories of patients according to their cardiovascular risk profile, therapeutic regimen, and clinical status and, finally, their overall risk status (e.g. ability to self-care). As indicated in the text above, it should be noted that clinic-based visits or interactive contacts using the latest remote technology can be substituted for home visits. Regardless of the mode of follow-up (i.e. personal versus remote contacts), the same principles for altering the frequency and intensity of chronic cardiac care, based on the patient profile and their immediate needs, should be strategically formulated and applied.

7.6 Promoting quality end-of-life

As discussed earlier, it is important to consider when it is appropriate to reconsider the goal of any therapeutic attempts to improve quality of life, avoid costly morbid events, and prolong survival, in favor of proactively promoting quality end-of-life. Whilst it is beyond the scope of this book to comprehensively describe the principles of palliation in the nonmalignant context it is worth considering the following.

Selecting patients for palliative care

There is strong argument for offering palliation to anyone who, in all probability, is likely to die within the next 12 months [22]. This obviates the need

Table 7.2 Schema for applying chronic cardiac care on an individual basis.

	Group 1 (symptom-free)				Group 2 (symptomatic)			
	A	B	C	D	A	B	C	D
Low risk	✓	✓			✓	✓		
Appropriately treated	✓		✓		✓		✓	
High risk			✓	✓			✓	✓
Inappropriately treated		✓		✓		✓		✓
Initial home visit within 1 week (72 hours)	✓	✓	✓	✓	✓	✓	✓	✓
Second home visit at 1–2 weeks	✓	✓	✓	✓	✓	✓	✓	✓
Routine 3 monthly phone calls	✓	✓	✓	✓	✓	✓	✓	✓
Weekly home visits for the first month	✓	✓	✓	✓	✓	✓	✓	✓
Weekly home visits extended for 1–2 months								✓
Weekly phone calls to reassess status				✓		✓	✓	✓
Monthly phone cafe to reassess health status			✓			✓		
Reapplication of service if readmitted	✓	✓	✓	✓	✓	✓	✓	✓

Key points
- All patients subject to a "safety net" of at least two home visits plus 3 monthly phone calls.
- Patients regularly reassessed and the amount of follow-up increased or reduced based on their clinical and psychosocial status.
- The specialist cardiac nurse's aim is to maximize the impact of initial intervention and limiting contact thereafter (excepting patient-initiated phone calls) with a focus on appropriate self-care behaviors.
- The management of patients who are either symptomatic and/or receiving inappropriate treatment after 3 months should be subject to an expert multidisciplinary review.
- The potential need for palliative care, as opposed to active management, should be strongly considered in those unlikely to survive beyond 12 months.

for a comprehensive review of all chronically ill patients. It is particularly important, therefore, for the specialist care nurse to remember to apply the principles of palliative care on the basis of "need" rather than "diagnosis". Clearly, extending palliation beyond malignancy raises a number of complex issues. Most health care professionals will be forced to overcome a natural desire to be optimistic and to avoid alarming patients unnecessarily with thoughts of impending death. It is in the best interests of the patient if the clinician does come to this difficult conclusion – even if the patient has not reached the same conclusion. Despite the problem of "denial" at the end-of-life, it is the frequent wish of patients that the doctor begins discussions about death [23]. There is, however, an inherent problem in predicting the illness trajectory of CHF and other forms of chronic cardiac disease. For example, in the SUP-PORT Study some patients with CHF had been predicted to have a greater than 50% chance of surviving six months, but died just three days later [24]. Not knowing how long the patient will live creates a situation of uncertainty that can, in theory, "paralyze" physicians and nurses alike: potentially preventing them from implementing palliative care [25]. In all probability there is no solution to such "treatment paralysis" without specific, professional guidelines and an increase in consumer expectations to prompt appropriate end-of-life care.

Applying palliative care in chronic cardiac disease

Fortunately, palliation encompasses a number of principles that can be applied quite effectively beyond malignancy using preexisting resources. Palliative care represents holistic management that has moved beyond medical cure. It focuses on the physical, psychological, social, and spiritual problems of the patient at the end of their life [23]. In simple terms, it equates to providing a good quality end to life by whatever means possible [22]. Although palliation has historically focussed on terminal malignancy, most people who are physically deteriorating and approaching the end-of-life experience similar problems. Four main issues are common to all patients who are expected to live less than 12 months:
• Deficits in basic self-care.
• Emotional distress.
• Pain and chronic symptoms.
• Malnutrition [25].
In CHF and chronic angina pectoris, persistent dyspnoea and chest pain, with associated limitations on all activities of daily living, is particularly distressing. Dealing with such problems requires a multidisciplinary approach combined with the core palliative care values of open and sensitive communication, a whole patient and carer approach, attention to symptom control and therapeutic dialogue.

7.7 Maintaining high standards: generating and analyzing audit data

As noted above, a comprehensive data set that is capable of tracking thera-peutic management, clinical status and key health outcomes is an important source of information on both an individual and service level. As such, it is extremely important to be able to monitor the performance of any service. The natural inclination is to assume that the results of any research are translated into clinical practice. This is, of course, a fallacy that is particularly true when one considers the nature of the intervention with its many "working parts", the variability in expertise in those who interact with patients and the need to incorporate new areas of practice. Unlike pharmacotherapy, specialist nurse-led management is not an exact science – in fact, it has a strong component of "art" as well as science.

The type of protocols and guidelines outlined in this book are an attempt to provide a uniformity of high standard of care. However, it important to audit health outcomes to ensure that a service is functioning as intended. Figure 7.4, representing audit data from the world-renowned Glasgow Heart Failure Nurse Liaison Service [26] demonstrates the utility of tracking impor-tant end-points to ensure that expected health outcomes (particularly when a specific intervention is applied across a range of institutions) are being met. As described in more detail in Chapter 4, on the basis of a meta-analysis of randomized studies of CHF management programs appear to prolong survival relative to usual care. [27] However, in the original study underpinning the Glasgow service [28] such prolonged survival was not observed.

However, as indicated by Figure 7.4, when audited and compared to ex-pected outcomes, patients recruited to the Glasgow CHF service have lower than expected 12-month survival rates [25]. Alternatively, the negative trial of increased access to primary care designed to improve outcomes in a range of

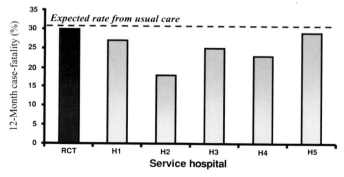

Figure 7.4 Expected versus actual 12-month mortality in CHF patients exposed to home-based, nurse-led management service in Glasgow, Scotland [25].

chronic disease states (including CHF) reported by Weinberger and colleagues [29], if anything, is a salient reminder that an intervention of this type, like any other medical or nursing "treatment," has the potential to lead to negative outcomes: particularly when issues of "operator dependence" and/or the "clinical cascade" whereby patient expectations rise and hospital admission thresholds decline, can adversely influence outcomes. Given a reasonable amount of time to be properly organized and the correct guidelines and protocols implemented, regular, independent auditing of the service's effectiveness should be undertaken. This auditing process should evaluate the service from a number of perspectives including the following:

- *Health care utilization.* A major aim of the service should be to reduce rehospitalization rates. Ideally, all rehospitalization occurring among those admitted to the recruiting hospital with a diagnosis of the target conditions (regardless of whether the patient was exposed to the service or not) should be monitored. If possible rehospitalization rates (at least over 6–12 months) should be compared to a previous period (for example, compared to a previous calendar year) and then compared on an accumulative basis thereafter. These comparisons can be made on an overall basis (all patients with chronic cardiac disease) and on the basis of exposure/nonexposure to the intervention. Making any comparison on this basis and with other hospitals is problematic without consideration of influencing variables other than the syndrome itself (for example, age, deprivation, comorbidity, and level of health care). The cost of these admissions should also be calculated.

- *Patient satisfaction and quality of life.* Whilst hospitalization rates are important, it is equally important to ensure that the intervention is making a positive impact on the patient's quality of life and satisfaction with their health care. A number of tools for measuring quality of life (both disease-specific and general health status questionnaires) are available for this purpose. Ideally, both of types of questionnaire should be used to measure changes in the patient's quality of life with additional consideration of their functional status (e.g. Canadian Heart and NYHA class plus results of six-minute walk test where appropriate). It is not necessary to audit every patient, but to generate a random sample from which measurements can be made. Measuring satisfaction with health care is much more problematic on a formal basis. It is possible, however, on an informal basis (for example, with a few well-directed questions) to gather useful information – as long as the mode of auditing is appropriate to the patient (for example, verbal questioning for older patients), allows for candid responses and is performed on an independent basis.

- *Family/carer satisfaction and quality of life.* Although family and carers are frequently identified as vital cogs in the management of chronic disease, they are often overlooked when an intervention (e.g. nurse-led CHF management) is applied on a research or service basis [30]. While an intervention may improve the quality of life of the individual with chronic cardiac disease, it is possible that those who care for that individual may be adversely affected by the fact that they have little or no respite from that burden of care. Moreover, they may be asked to take a greater role than before; something that may be too onerous for an older partner, for example, who also suffers from chronic illness. As such, family and carers should always be included in the auditing process!

- *Survival.* As discussed previously, optimal chronic cardiac care has the potential to prolong survival rates. Alternatively, given narrow risk-benefits associated with many therapeutic agents (e.g. anticoagulation and antiarrhythmic therapy in AF and spironolactone in CHF) there is a potential for mismanagement to adversely impact on patient survival.

7.8 Creating a harmonious health care team

Whilst it is possible to control many of the facets of day-to-day management of the patient with chronic cardiac disease and their contact with specialist staff, it is vital to create a productive and harmonious relationship with other members of the health care team. Based on the concept of the "weakest link" it is easy to see how negative outcomes generated from the type of auditing process described above could be derived from factors outside of the control of the nurse-led, chronic cardiac care team. A number of key processes need to be undertaken on a proactive basis to minimize the risk of poor health outcomes in this context:

- *Creating a "partnership" with hospital staff.* In the initial stages of developing a new service it is especially important to spend time explaining exactly what will be happening and why the service will be of benefit to those members of the health care system who are affected by it. For those hospital-based health professionals who come into contact with potential candidates for the new service, it should be openly acknowledged that their workload would be (initially at least) increased. However, by assisting the specialist cardiac nurse to identify and then refer eligible patients for the service and then gather appropriate information and ensure appropriate discharge planning, they are likely to reduce their workload in the longer-term. In the first few months of the service therefore, the specialist nurse needs to spend a good deal of time creating a partnership with hospital staff – in essence becoming part of the furniture! With this partnership firmly cemented it should be possible to implement the following type of protocol for identifying and recruiting patients.

- *Creating a harmonious relationship with community-based services.* The same principles that were used to ensure a harmonious relationship with hospital staff and services should also be applied to ensure the same sort of relationship with the community-based health care professionals. Obviously, considering the diversity and breadth of these it will be inherently more difficult to achieve. Once again, however, it is important to identify who will be most affected by the service and to convince them that it will be of overall benefit to them and, most importantly the patient. Clearly, the most important health care professional to consider is the general practitioner. In this respect, dealing with these health care professionals on an organizational level is advantageous in spreading the broader message and providing information about the service. In order to attain a trusting and an effective relationship, however, it is advisable to take the time on an individual level to inform and clarify points of issue with each patient's community-based physician: another good reason for gradually building up the service! Having firmly established guidelines/protocols that are agreed upon by the major stakeholders and specifying the exact role of the specialist cardiac heart failure nurse will facilitate this process.

Clearly, positive health outcome data (typically derived from independently derived audit data that is consistent with expected benefits) is the most powerful and compelling reason for initially skeptical or recalcitrant health care professionals (and indeed potential patients) to collaborate and further improve the cost-efficiencies of the newly introduced program/service.

7.9 Successfully implementing well-made plans

Introducing any intervention of this type as a formal program or service is not easy without key personnel who are experienced in implementing and budgeting for new health care services. As indicated by Figure 7.2, there is an obvious need for sufficient funding and support to provide the specialist cardiac nurse with both equipment and time to develop and implement effective protocols. With or without sufficient funding, however, the service will undoubtedly fail without the support of key personnel. As such, the optimal amount of support will include that of leading cardiologists, general practitioners/primary care physicians, health care administrators, and nurses at the local, regional, or national level where appropriate.

Prior to patient recruitment we would suggest a final review of the service development process to ensure that all the following steps have been undertaken, or at least considered:

1 Develop precise and realistic aims and objectives for the service.
2 Establish close links with both the hospital and community-based health care services.
3 Establish concise and realistic inclusion criteria for those patients eligible to receive the service.
4 Establish precise protocols for the identification and recruitment of patients with chronic cardiac disease.
5 Establish precise protocols for the immediate postdischarge care of the patient (including the coordination of health care and the management of pharmacological and nonpharmacological treatment strategies).
6 Establish precise protocols for the longer-term management of the patient – according to their risk of rehospitalization and overall health care needs.

7 Establish comprehensive and independent auditing procedures.

8 Make a comprehensive list of infrastructure and equipment needs ensuring that all items and service requirements are carefully accounted for.

9 Recruit the specialist cardiac nurses using strict selection criteria, ensuring that the appointed personnel are adequately paid and are subject to a rigorous and comprehensive training program.

10 Introduce the service slowly allowing time for protocols to be tested properly and any teething problems are adequately addressed.

In order to facilitate future developments of this kind in other regions and countries, it would be extremely useful for a "blueprint" of the developed service to be available for interested parties to obtain and consider via a dedicated web site or publication.

7.10 Summary

As can be appreciated, not withstanding the growing evidence and experience relating to nurse-led, CHF management programs, the establishment of cost-effective programs of nurse-led chronic cardiac care represents an evolving field of endeavor. Fortunately, as outlined above, there are an eclectic range of principles and theories of management that provide a good framework for applying cost-effective chronic cardiac care. In the next 5–10 years, there will no doubt be much more evidence (both in terms of health outcomes and practical strategies) to guide the management of chronic cardiac care into the 21st Century.

References

1 Clark RA, Driscoll A, Nottage J, et al. Overcoming the tyranny of distance: a mismatch of supply and demand for specialist chronic heart failure management in Australia. *Heart Lung & Circulation* 2005; **14 (S1)**: S112.

2 Stewart S, Blue L, Walker A, et al. An economic analysis of specialist heart failure management in the UK – can we afford not to implement it? *Eur Heart J* 2002; **23**:1369–1378.

3 Stewart S. The cost of caring for chronic heart failure. *Eur J Heart Failure* 2005; **16**:423–428.

4 International Council of Nurses (2003). *Definition and characteristics for nurse practitioner/advanced practice nursing roles.* http://www.icn-apnetwork.org: Retrieved April 20, 2004.

5 Brown S, Grimes D. A meta-analysis of nurse practitioners and nurse midwives in primary care. *Nur Res* 1995; **44**:332–339.

6 Dunn L. A literature review of advanced clinical nursing practice in the United States of America. *J Adv Nur* 1995; **25**:814–819.

7 Edmunds MV (2003). *Nurse practitioners: Remembering the past, planning the future.* http://www.medscape.com/viewarticle/408388print: Accessed June 2004.

8 Pearson LJ. Annual update of how each state stands on legislative issues affecting advanced nursing practice. *Nur Pract* 1999; **24**:16–83.

9 Read S, Roberts-Davis M, Gilbert P. *Preparing to work together: seeking consensus on nursepractitioner roles and programmes in England.* Melbourne, Australia: Abstract presented at 6th International Nurse Practitioner Conference, 1998.

10 Horrocks S, Anderson E, Salisbury C. Systematic review of whether nurse practitioners working in primary care can provide equivalent care to doctors. *Br Med J* 2002; **324**:819–823.

11 Pearson S, Inglis SC, McLennan S, et al. Prolonged effects of a home-based intervention in chronically ill patients. *Arch Intern Med* – Accepted for publication (2005).

12 Stewart S, Blue L, eds. *Specialist Nurse Intervention in Chronic Heart Failure: from research to practice.* London: BMJ Books, 2004.

13 Charlson ME, Pompei P, Ales KL, MacKenzie CR. A new method of classifying prognostic comorbidity in longitudinal studies: development and validation. *J Chron Dis* 1987; **40**:373–383.

14 Folstein MF, Folstein SE, McHugh PR. Mini-mental state: a practical method for grading the cognitive state of patients for the clinician. *J Psychiat Res* 1975; **12**:189–198.

15 Devlin N, Hansen P, Herbison P, Macran S. A new and improved EQ-5D valuation questionnaire? Results from a pilot study. *Eur J Health Econ* 2005; **6**:73–82.

16 McHorney C, Ware JE, Lu JF, Sherbourne CD. The MOS 36-item short form health survey (SF-36): Psychometric and clinical tests of validity in measuring physical and mental health constructs. *Med Care* 1994; **32**:551–567.

17 Rector TS, Kubo SH, Cohn JN. Validity of the Minnesota living with heart failure questionnaire as a measure of therapeutic response to enalapril of placebo. *Am J Cardiol* 1993; **71**:1106–1107.

18 Cameron J, Worral-Carter L, New G, Driscoll A, Stewart S. Extent of Heart Failure Self-Care as an Endpoint to Patient Education: A Review of the Literature: Submitted for publication.

19 Riegel B, Carlson B, Glaser D. Development and testing of a clinical tool measuring self-management of heart failure. *Heart & Lung* 2000; **29**(91):4–15.

20 Carlson B, Riegel B, Moser D. Self-care abilities of patients with heart failure. *Heart & Lung,* 2001; **30**(5):351–359.

21 Clark NM, Gong M. Management of chronic disease by practitioners and patients: are we teaching the wrong things? *BMJ* 2000; **320**:572–575.

22 McMurray JJV, Stewart S. Palliative care for heart failure? *Br Med J* 2002; **325**:915–916.

23 Gore JM, Brophy GJ, Greenstone MA. How well do we care for patients with end stage chronic obstructive pulmonary disease (COPD)? A comparison of palliative care and quality of life in COPD and lung cancer. *Thorax* 2000; **55**:1000–1006.

24 Levenson JW, McCarthy EP, Lynn J, et al. The last six months of life for patients with congestive heart failure. *J Am Geriatr Soc* 2000; **48**:S101–S109.

25 Goodlin SJ, Jette AM, Lynn J, Wasson JH. Community physicians describe management issues for patients expected to live less than twelve months. *J Palliat Care* 1998; **14**:30–35.

26 Russell K, Freeman A, Blue L, Stewart S. A blueprint for identifying and managing patients within a heart failure service. In: Stewart S, Blue L, eds. *Specialist Nurse Intervention in Chronic Heart Failure: from research to practice.* London: BMJ Books, 2004.

27 McAlister FA, Stewart S, Ferrua S, McMurray JJ. Multidisciplinary strategies for the management of heart failure patients at high risk for admission: a systematic review of randomized trials. *J Am Coll Cardiol* 2004; **44**:810–819.
28 Blue L, Strong E, Murdoch DR, et al. Improving long-term outcome with specialist nurse intervention in heart failure: a randomized trial. *BMJ* 2002; **323**:1112–1115.
29 Oddone EZ, Weinberger M, Giobbie-Hurder A, et al. Enhanced access to primary care for patients with congestive heart failure. Veterans affairs cooperative study group on primary care and hospital readmission. *Eff Clin Pract* 1999; **2**:201–209.
30 Stewart S. Recognising the "other half" of the heart failure equation: are we doing enough for family caregivers? *Eur J Heart Fail* 2005; **7**:590–591.

Index

Note: page numbers in *italics* represent figures, those in **bold** represent tables.